SORAYA

A Life of Music,
a Legacy of Hope

SORAYA

FOREWORD BY NANCY G. BRINKER
FOUNDER, SUSAN G. KOMEN FOR THE CURE®

BICENTENNIAL
1807
WILEY
2007
BICENTENNIAL

John Wiley & Sons, Inc.

A hero does not have to win.
A hero does not have to be larger than life.
A hero can be an ordinary person who overcomes
Extraordinary events with dignity and grace.

—Soraya

It was Soraya's wish that her proceeds from this book go to breast cancer awareness and education programs.

For more information about Soraya and her mission, and to find out other ways you can help, visit www.Soraya.com.

CONTENTS

Foreword *by Nancy G. Brinker*   vii

A Labor of Love: Publishing Soraya's Story *by Joyce Fleming*   xi

Preface   xv

PART ONE
THE ROOTS

Chapter 1	Gifts	3
Chapter 2	The Fabric of Courage	8
Chapter 3	Riches and Rag Dolls	11
Chapter 4	A Tradition of Silence	17
Chapter 5	A Struggle to Survive, a Surplus of Love	22
Chapter 6	Mother and Daughter	33
	Memories	41

PART TWO
THE RISE

Chapter 7	Solo Mi Dios	59
Chapter 8	Music Lessons	67
Chapter 9	Heights and Depths	75

Chapter 10	How Do I?	83
Chapter 11	An Army for Change	91
Chapter 12	Reborn	99
	Memories	109

PART THREE
THE RACE

Chapter 13	Miracles, Large and Small	161
Chapter 14	Signs of Life	169
Chapter 15	Singing to the Angels	179
	Memories	187

Epilogue *by Itzel Diaz*	219
Inspirations: Eleven Helpful Themes *interpreted and compiled by Joyce Fleming and Alison Provost*	225
A Medical Note *by Joyce O'Shaughnessy, M.D.*	238
Photo Credits	240

FOREWORD

BY NANCY G. BRINKER
founder, Susan G. Komen for the Cure®

I'll never forget the first time I met her. Soraya was performing at a fund-raiser for a Spanish television network in her beloved Miami. As it did everywhere, her spirit filled the room. True to her name, she was a shining star, stunning in her beauty and inspiring in her sincerity.

But it was what she said to me offstage that revealed the larger mission of her life and music. "Let me help you educate Hispanic women," she said, speaking of breast cancer, the disease that had taken her grandmother, her mother, and soon, her aunt—her *angelitos*, as she called them.

Soraya wasn't a performer looking for attention. She was a daughter, a niece, and a granddaughter looking to make a difference. She knew that Latinas are less likely than other women to perform breast self-exams and to have regular clinical checkups and yearly mammograms. As a result, Latinas tend to be diagnosed at a later, more advanced stage, making them more likely to die from breast cancer.

But Soraya also knew that when breast cancer is caught early, before it spreads beyond the breast, the five-year survival rate is greater than 95 percent. "Everyone deserves a fighting chance to survive this terrible disease," she often said.

To help give Latinas that chance, those of us at the Susan G. Komen Breast Cancer Foundation (now the Susan G. Komen for the Cure) worked with Soraya to include information about breast health and the importance of early detection in her next album, *Cuerpo y Alma / I'm Yours.*

A few months later, the phone rang. It was Soraya. She was in Colombia caring for her aunt. "Nancy, I found a lump," she said. Within days, her doctors had confirmed the worst—Stage 3 breast cancer, one of the most aggressive forms of the disease.

It was all too familiar, like the unforgettable phone call I received nearly thirty years ago from my sister, Susan G. Komen. Like Susan, Soraya was diagnosed young—Susan at thirty-three, Soraya at thirty-one. Both had their whole lives ahead of them. And both made a promise—a solemn vow to end this disease and to spare other women the pain and loss they had endured.

In the few years that followed, Soraya's life, like her lyrics, became an inspiration. As she wrote so poignantly in "No One Else"/"Por Ser Quien Soy":

> *With an army in my soul, soldiers of love, warriors of faith*
> *Fighting a battle against the enemy with no face*
>
> .   .   .   .
>
> *In my darkest hour, when I could barely see*
> *I found the essence of a woman I never dreamed I could be*

Some suggested that she not discuss her disease in public, that doing so would undermine her image. But with compassion, love, and courage, Soraya went public. And after it seemed she had beaten the cancer, she shared the darkest hours of her fight, empowering women, especially Latinas, to overcome the silence and shame that so often prevents women from seeking the early treatment that saves lives.

As a singer-songwriter, she blended the traditions and influences of many Latin cultures. As Komen's "Latin Ambassador," her love, honesty, and humility (appearing often without her hair) transcended countries, cultures, and language and touched the hearts of millions.

At Komen, we will remain forever grateful to Soraya. She was not only an eloquent spokeswoman whose words and wisdom moved audiences to tears and to action. She was a beloved friend who made us better, helping us clarify and carry our message of hope to a new generation of Spanish-speaking women. Those women now look to her with the same love and awe that Soraya felt for her own mother when she sang, "I think of how strong you were and it helps me to get by."

Soraya never stopped teaching us, not even in the darkest hours when her cancer returned. As she neared the end of her journey, Soraya, as always, reached into her soul and found just the right words to capture her spirit: "I know there are many questions without answers, and that hope doesn't leave with me. . . . My mission does not end with my physical story."

And that, I believe, will be the greatest legacy of her life—the hope she gave, the hearts she touched, and the lives she saved. Soraya left us far, far too early. But like her angelic voice that moved us all, her music and her mission live on.

A LABOR OF LOVE
PUBLISHING SORAYA'S STORY

BY JOYCE FLEMING
Soraya's manager

Soraya was always a writer. The world knew her as an award-winning *songwriter*, but she always wrote. She almost always had a pencil or pen in her hand. She wrote on napkins and on the covers of the current book she was reading; she wrote poetry, essays, articles. She was always inspirational and motivational, but careful never to impose her ideas. Until, that is, she was diagnosed with breast cancer.

So it wasn't out of character that in 2001, during her breast cancer treatments, Soraya began to write a book. Her intention at that time was to share the story of strength and courage of the women in her family who had endured so much. Shortly after preparing an outline and signing with a literary agent, she put the writing down. She said, "Who am I to write a book? I am a songwriter, and I will keep to what I do best. Besides, who would be interested in my story anyway?"

In 2003, she recorded and produced her fourth record, *Soraya*, her after-cancer "comeback" album. Her message was loud and clear: "Fight for your life, you deserve it." The years to follow were filled with incredible moments of revelation and joy. Soraya was back on top and immensely enjoying her new life.

In 2005, she began promoting her fifth album. But unfortunately, the cancer had returned with a vengeance. Even though she considered it to be in a state of controlled remission, her life was changed. The concept of time was suddenly very present, and we carefully planned her schedule to allow her the best quality of life. This time, she kept her illness very quiet because, as she says in this memoir, she had something to prove. She needed to prove that with today's medicine and with a controlled, focused mind one can live with cancer. So she performed as before in front of thousands, traveled, visited radio stations, went on TV, met with medical professionals, attended fundraising events, and lent her voice to many great people who are doing great things to eradicate breast cancer as a life-threatening disease.

Still, unbeknownst to almost everyone, she was very, very sick. And yet, always smiling.

In late November 2005 she decided it was time to go home, enjoy her family and dear friends, and pursue the most aggressive treatments. She was confident she would knock the cancer back into full remission. That is when she decided that now was the time to write a book. She found her muse and sat with her computer, indoors, outdoors, in her garden, by her pool. Wherever she wanted or needed to be in order for the words to flow, she went. This time she was clear: until she could get better, this would be the best way for her to communicate her message, and she had a perfect plan. She would interview her aunts and uncle, get the facts straight, and put the story down, and we would release this book. She wrote day and night. She was on a mission.

In late February 2006, she called me to say, "It's done, my work is done, now it's your turn, your work must begin." She then passed out three copies of her first draft to get initial feedback. We all agreed that one way or another we would get this book into people's hands. And we would market it, with Soraya there to promote it.

Soraya was a perfectionist, and she didn't believe she was done—not with the book, and not with her life. But her team at the marketing firm PowerPact was anxious to figure out what kind of product they'd be promoting, and so she finally agreed to turn over the manuscript. Soraya had kept the severity of her illness from everyone but me and a couple of her closest friends, and it was only through the book draft that her friends at PowerPact found out just how ill she was. Rose Ann Domenici, a managing director there, and Alison Provost, PowerPact's CEO, quickly read the manuscript and called me, shocked and in tears.

When she handed over her book, Soraya made her instructions very clear: do whatever it takes to get it published, and donate the profits to breast cancer education and awareness initiatives. Alison got right down to editing, and within a day or two she had pages of questions for Soraya. Day by day we kept hoping there'd be a good time for Soraya to answer those questions, but it was not to be. Soraya died about ten days after we began our work. Answers would ultimately have to come from Soraya's loved ones, and whatever holes she had inadvertently left in her story were carefully researched and filled in by those of us who knew her best, without changing her style and her intentions.

But beyond editing Soraya's work, we wanted to add some pieces to Soraya's book. She had become an incredibly powerful public speaker, and her speeches featured strong themes of hope and empowerment. She often asked, "If we were to summarize these things I say into actionable advice, what would that look like?" We reviewed her speeches and writings, pulled out the major themes, gave them names and descriptions, and added this inspirational material at the end of the book. (In this edition, this section, newly arranged, is titled "Inspirations: Eleven Helpful Themes.")

We also enlisted Dr. Joyce O'Shaughnessy to write a medical note to reassure women that Soraya's breast cancer is not typical. Dr. O, as she is known, is one of the world's leading breast cancer practitioners, responsible for large bodies of significant research. She became an ally of Soraya's and helped move her mission forward. We're grateful to her.

When Soraya posted a good-bye letter to her fans on her Web site, she mentioned that she was leaving behind a memoir. As a result, there was interest from several publishers. We accepted an offer from Grupo Editorial Norma, a major Latin American publisher in Colombia. In September 2006, *Con Las Cuerdas Rotas* (Broken Strings) hit the shelves in the Spanish-speaking world. It has since gone into its third printing and has broken records for Spanish-language books. Just before the release of that book, we were invited by our friends at Yoplait to present Soraya and her work to the U.S. publisher John Wiley & Sons. Wiley immediately understood the need to publish this work and began to advise us on how to get it done.

Most importantly, the publisher wanted us to add more details about Soraya's life. This created a dilemma. After all the care we had taken in the editing to not add anything extraneous to what Soraya intended to be her story, we certainly couldn't write new material for her. But the truth is that we were thrilled to have a reason to tell more of her story, and we decided to do so by creating scrapbook-like sections that illustrate all she had accomplished as a musician, a cancer survivor, and a breast cancer education advocate. Alison, Itzel Diaz (Soraya's best friend), and I gathered scores of photos and asked Soraya's friends, relatives, coworkers, and fans to write captions and stories that would help fill in the blanks. The resulting new sections, titled "Memories," appear at the end of each of the parts of this book.

As hard as it has been for all of us to re-live the precious time we had with her, each and every person we contacted had another amazing Soraya story to add to our collection of memories. It was just more proof that Soraya was not only a great daughter, aunt, niece, and granddaughter, and a great friend to so many, she was also an inspiration to everyone who met her.

This book was a genuine labor of love for Soraya, and if ever there was a dying wish, getting it published and funding more educational programs with its proceeds was Soraya's. She should be proud of what she wrote, and surely she's smiling now at all the heartfelt contributions her friends and family have made to the book.

We hope that *Soraya: A Life of Music, a Legacy of Hope* inspires you, whether you're healthy and thriving or struggling to get through a difficult time.

PREFACE

This is not my autobiography. I am much too young to think that I have completed my cycle. I am not so vain as to believe that my entire life is so important that it beckons to be shared. In the following pages, I will present to you pieces of my life. They are parts that I feel are worthy to be shared because they are both utterly personal and yet hauntingly universal.

I have delicately chosen what to share and as I have done throughout my entire public career, I have chosen what to keep as my own. There are many people—family, friends, fans, and colleagues—who have been an integral part of my life. My omission of them is purposeful and in no way lessens their importance to me.

In spite of the tragedies that run like a river through my lifeline, it has miraculously been a life filled with joy and love. In both my personal and professional lives I have achieved what most only dream. It is this sweet taste of happiness that has kept me going and has spurred a drive that has never allowed me to give up.

This narrative is not a medical reference, nor is it meant to be a source of information about breast cancer. I hope it will serve as a guide toward hope and an inspiration for those who are losing their balance. I do not have a Ph.D. in psychology, philosophy, or theology. My qualifications to write this book are simple. I am a woman who has lived more than an ordinary life. Every day I have made an effort to not simply pass the time but to relish it and try to be a better human being than I was just a few minutes ago. My goal has been to connect with my ever-changing truths and to live a life worth living. With or without cancer, we all struggle with issues of mortality, family history, and our own legacy. We confront ego, society, religion, love, and our own demons. It is the shared human experience. This narrative is meant to remind us that even in the bleakest hour of our lives, there is always, hidden as it might be sometimes, a reason to keep on believing. Working our way toward a reunion with our inner self is the only accomplishment worthy of our undivided attention. It is the fuel for all of our dreams and hopes.

PART ONE
THE ROOTS

Chapter 1

GIFTS

*P*ain has been scorched into every fiber of my being. Sometimes, in the right light, it grows so large that I see its shadow, haunting me, reminding me of all I have lost. But I have learned to coexist with the bruises and scars, with the mind-numbing aches, and with the lonely throbbing in that vast, black space deep within my soul. I know every turn of its jagged corners, how frightening it is to teeter dangerously over its edge. Yet I never allow myself to look down; I can only try to keep the pain from getting any deeper and to keep from falling into its abyss.

I always knew that I was disciplined, but I never knew how strong was the blind courage that ran in my blood. I never doubted, or listened to those who said I would fail. I might come out on the other side beaten and banged up, but I let nothing stand in my way. Somehow I find a way to persevere. Those were the gifts I had from the start. But until I watched my mother die, I never understood what it meant to love and to be loved. Until I learned of my grandmother's story of loss and new beginnings, I didn't understand dignity. I came to know faith and charity through the life of my mother's eldest sister, my *tia* America, who faced every setback with an unwavering calm and not an ounce of self-pity. And until I, too, became ill with the disease that will forever bind all four of us, I never understood why I had been given this gift to find hope in the most desolate places of the heart.

I am a singer, songwriter, musician, and producer. I have toured the world with my music, been on countless magazine covers, and have met and performed with some of my greatest idols, the people who've shaped my musical identity. My studio office walls are lined with gold records and awards, and in the last several years I have become a fervent patient advocate and public speaker. But those are not my proudest accomplishments in life. For I am also the granddaughter, niece, and daughter of three women who died from breast cancer, and I write these words today as a woman who has survived a diagnosis of advanced breast cancer beyond her projected years. It is not the sum of these years that emboldens my stride, but rather how I have redefined my concepts of time, quality of life, and all of the things in between.

The lives of my mother, my grandmother, and my aunt are the prologue to my own story. Through their example, they taught me what it means to be alive. From them I have inherited the courage to carry on through the incomprehensible with dignity and love. They taught me how to live when life itself is filled with uncertainties and the truth of certain death becomes undeniable. But also, they left me a complex legacy that challenges me both physically and emotionally, as they chose such completely different paths for confronting their illness that I often feel they left me with no clear choice as to which path is best. They faced daunting challenges beyond the cancer, and it is this struggle that has illuminated my own path: they taught me how to sort through the particles of life and only grab onto what really matters. Their physical confrontations with this disease were horrific, yet their spiritual growth throughout the suffering would make a believer out of the staunchest skeptic. I found something extraordinary in these ordinary women, and through them I have found myself. Their lives have served as a chronicle for mine.

As I look through family photos, I see beyond the disease that ties us together forever in our family's story, and I find my own eyes warmly looking back at me in the gaze of my mother's mother, my *abuela* Nayibe (nye-EE-bay). Headstrong and full of life, my grandmother left her war-torn homeland of Lebanon at age nine with her recently widowed mother, Jamile (jah-MEE-lay), and her grandmother, Mercedes. They set out on a steamship across the Mediterranean and ultimately the Atlantic with no certain plans and only a vague image of the place where they would disembark and start anew. Later in life, long after she had settled in Colombia, my *abuela* Nayibe would face the primitive treatments available to women of her generation who had "tumors." She died long before I was born, but Nayibe was the first in line to bravely face our fate, and she became an unwitting role model.

I have a collection of memories of my *tia* America, Nayibe's oldest daughter. I wanted to be her ever since I was old enough to walk. My aunt was regal and beautiful, and she stepped up to be the family matriarch after my grandmother, Nayibe, died. *Tia* America's life was filled with obstacles—tragedies that would easily destroy a person of a lesser constitution. But she carried on and took care of not only her own family but also all of us, even throughout her problematic life and her cancer diagnosis. Until the end, she was still the one in control. She was still the one with words of encouragement. Yes, if her fate is to be mine, I want to be her.

And then, of course, there is my mom, Yamila (yah-MEE-la), Nayibe's fourth child and America's little sister.

"Sorayita," I remember her calling out for me. But through the years of silence after her death, her voice is getting harder and harder to remember. Before she became my mom, a young Yamila followed her husband to pursue the American Dream. Just as her mother, Nayibe, had left Lebanon, my mother, too, left behind all she knew in Colombia and arrived in a new world. As the years passed, she went from being a shy and quiet young woman who sought company in books to one who spoke her mind and surrounded herself with friends and laughter. After her cancer diagnosis, she fought with unnerving strength. However, she was forever changed. The treatment abruptly removed much more than her tumors. But somehow she kept going. Her inner light changed colors, but it never dimmed. Even when the doctors lost hope, she still held on. Of all the ways I came to emulate her, surely she hoped that this ability to hold on was the one lesson that I would never need to use.

Fortunately, since my diagnosis and consequent perpetual battle with this disease, I have searched my heritage and pulled from it the strength of these amazing women. I saw them bravely endure the treatments that were not so targeted as they are now. I saw them live alongside uncertainty with unwavering courage. Yet the greatest lesson of all came from their confrontation with, and ultimate acceptance of, their own mortality. As with all of us who lose a loved one, the time we had together was not enough, but for the most part, it was well spent. My *abuela* Nayibe, my *tia* America, and my mom all died with peace in their hearts. But they also spent much time battling both the physical pain of the disease and the heartbreaking realization that they would be leaving their children behind. The examples they set have helped me manage a wave of emotions through my battle with breast cancer. If I were to lose my focus even for a second, the tide would pull me out and I would sink, self-pity shackled to my ankles like lead weights. The experiences of my relatives have helped me to live at a heightened level, all the while proving the medical statistics wrong. With all I was told I might not ever do again, with all the time I was told I might not have, my ears remained deaf to these proclamations, and my mind pushed, and still pushes, my body to stay strong and carry on. Every day I move, walk, sing, speak, breathe, and live with the energy that my three *angelitos* left behind for me.

I have committed my life to living my life, concentrating all the while on balancing life-extending treatments with life-enhancing living. The reality of this disease will not be an impediment but rather a tool I use to harvest more out of the time I have been given—and maybe even the time I wasn't meant to have. I have become a professional patient, determined not to let it alter the quality of my existence. This is my reality and I do not fight it anymore. I choose to exert my energy living the life that, thanks to today's treatments, those who came before me never had the opportunity to enjoy.

I will keep on singing, and I will keep on sharing my message. I will continue on my mission to share hope not with empty words but rather by serving as a multidimensional example of what it means to be alive. I refuse to fall victim to a limited definition of self. It is this more enlightened woman that I present in this book, with the hope that others can recognize in me pieces of themselves, just as I saw my reflection in my *abuela* Nayibe, my *tia* America, and my mom.

The chronicle must end with me.

I stand at the end of the line, holding on firmly to the parts of the tradition worth holding on to, shattering those that are not, and living every day with the belief that maybe I will be the one to finally break the legacy. Maybe I will be able to grow old. If not, at least let me enjoy the ride to its fullest. Starting every day by waking up to your own mortality teaches one how fragile it all is. Each moment is treasured as if it were the last. And when I stumble and get tangled and feel I cannot bear any more, I reach deep within and run my hands through the ashes at the bottom of my soul. I am aware of what that dust once was, emergent but carefree. But I also know that from this rubble I will once again rebuild myself. I will rise like the women who preceded me. Time and time again, if need be, I will be a phoenix, and my new song will be sweeter than the last.

Chapter 2

THE FABRIC OF COURAGE

*M*ine is a family that for as long as we can remember has been run by women—women who learned to find strange comfort in even the most hellish of circumstances. In the middle of my exploration into my own identity, I had to stop and understand where I came from in order to better comprehend where I stood and how I was going to define my own troubled destiny. I'm thankful to have come from a culture where holding on to our history is sacrosanct. Perhaps this is an old-world sensibility, as it seems not so common in the United States, but for me, these women sketched a diagram showing not merely how to cope but how to thrive. My mother's stories began with Mercedes and Jamile, women who were the epitome of female leadership and independence, and women who set a brisk pace for the rest of us to follow.

Armed with the basics, an innate street savvy, and a stockpile of courage, a precocious nine-year-old named Nayibe boarded the over-crowded steamship. It was 1925, in Lebanon. Holding on tightly to her mother Jamile's hand and comforted by the familiar plume of smoke from her grandmother Mercedes' cigarette, she stepped onto this floating, mysterious, unknown world.

Hundreds of families were pushing and sliding their way through the tight corners of the large ship on their way to makeshift cabins. They brought whatever they could carry, and even before setting sail, the bartering had begun. Olives and figs were traded for cigarettes and textiles. They were all erroneously given Turkish passports by the government that had pushed them out onto this sea, and together, this mass exodus of "Turkos," as they would incorrectly be labeled in their new homeland, set off to a faraway place called Colombia. Behind them remained farms, homes, relatives, and broken dreams. On the horizon awaited a new beginning. Few of them spoke Spanish.

The melodic sounds of Arabic and French filled the hallways of the ship as the women found their way into the galleys to prepare the kibbes, meat-filled patties that are a Lebanese specialty, and tabouli, a bulgur wheat salad served with pita or lettuce, for their temporary extended families. Like so many other women widowed by the war of independence and the creation of Lebanon in 1920, my great-grandmother Jamile and my great-great-grandmother Mercedes had been widowed as well. They had both seen the men of their family fall under a shower of bullets or die from illnesses contracted during the war. Religious persecution was at a peak. This matriarchal family of Christians had witnessed enough horrors, and the women had decided they would not wait for more bloodshed to take even more lives.

Fleeing the violence with young Nayibe in tow, they drew from their mercantile blood and sold most of what they had. They kept their cash in crisp, white handkerchiefs that, for the rest of both Mercedes' and Jamile's lives, would be placed underneath their bra straps even while they slept. What little they had not sold they packed into an elaborate wood- and leather-bound trunk. Their belongings consisted of a copper and silver bed, jewelry, food, an armoire, and a few household items. Fortunately, Mercedes had done well and was able to accumulate substantial capital by selling her land and her textile store in Lebanon. From her successes they knew they had enough to make the trip and get settled in Colombia, but they prayed that they would have enough to start new income-producing ventures once they got there.

The women had taken control of their destiny. Failure was not an option. Even by today's standards, theirs was quite a feat for any woman to undertake. I can only imagine the myriad emotions they must have felt, the sadness of leaving all they had ever known coupled with the liberating anticipation of a new beginning in a brand new world. I learned a lot from hearing my mother and my aunts tell the stories of these brave, adventuresome women. It tells me that more than illness got passed along through the generations. Their invincible spirit made it through, too, and I know my independent attitude comes from them.

But still, the journey was difficult for Mercedes, Jamile, and Nayibe. The seas were rough, and bad weather seemed to be an everyday occurrence. But hard times were all these three had ever known, and there was never a moment to complain or to worry. The older women would continuously clean their quarters, and upon nightfall the ship would grow dark and they would pass the time sharing stories about their homeland, stories about those they lost and why they chose to leave. Turning over a small coffee cup onto its saucer, the older women would read the fortunes of willing subjects in the designs left by the coffee grounds. They would crack an egg into water and create elaborate destinies based on the forms it would take. Later on, my mom would entertain me with this same "magic," and now I find myself cracking eggs with my godchildren so that I might tell their fortunes as well.

As the monotony of sea travel began to take hold of these first-time pilgrims, young Nayibe would dream: What would their new home look like? How do girls dress in this new world? Like most of the females in my family, Nayibe knew that with hard work they would get by and surely create happiness along the way. But every morning with the first light of day, Nayibe's nighttime reveries would come to an abrupt halt when Mercedes would give her granddaughter a long list of tasks to accomplish. Every day it was the same routine, until one spectacular morning nine weeks later.

Chapter 3

RICHES AND
RAG DOLLS

*F*inally the ship approached port, and the three women, along with hundreds of others, set foot on the shores of Buenaventura, Colombia, just south of the Panama Canal, which had been completed eleven years earlier.

Armed with old traditions and eyes hardened by war, they were quite a sight to behold. Mercedes was in mourning and dressed only in black, from her undergarments and stockings to her dress and her ballet-type slippers. Her clothing reflected not only tradition but also the status of her heart. Her blue eyes and light hair, always styled in a single long braid, created quite a contrast. Colombian immigration officials processed them, and they immediately set off for Cali, the city that to this day is home for my family.

This mass exodus from Lebanon had been going on from the 1880s and continued until about 1930. Many Christian Lebanese were swindled at their port of embarkation in the Ottoman Empire. After paying their fare, they realized only after their arrival that they were not in

Colombia, where they had a relative or friend waiting for them, but in Brazil, cheated of the passage around the northern coast of South America. Others ended up in a strange place called New York. But for the ones whose voyage did not go awry, they were outsiders in Colombia until their hard work and resourcefulness proved fruitful not only for them but for the country as a whole. Many changed their names upon arrival. Some did it on purpose to fit in, and others were simply the victim of the human error of an immigration officer who was unable to correctly spell these unfamiliar new names. My family's surname stayed the same—Garib (gah-REEB). The tradition of honoring our Middle Eastern heritage with Arabic names continued with my own name. Soraya (so-RYE-yah), depending on the Arabic dialect, represents a constellation of stars. More poetically, it is a light in the night sky.

The arrival of war refugees stirred up commerce and industry in Colombia, this oldest of the Latin American democracies. Textile trading, money exchanges, accounting offices, bakeries, restaurants, clothing manufacturing, cattle ranching, and agriculture were all stimulated by this new segment of the society. Even the import of the first automobile into Colombia in 1912 is credited to a "Syrian Lebanese" immigrant.

As for my family, together they stepped onto Colombian soil and silently vowed to rely on no one but themselves. Mercedes and Jamile knew how to make something from nothing. Whereas some of their travel companions might have been in survival mode, unable to do more than live moment to moment, these women, with a deeply ingrained sense of entrepreneurship, were already looking beyond tomorrow to find the path to a good and prosperous life. They invested all they brought on that long sea voyage into their new lives, and they invested well.

Born a merchant, Mercedes chain-smoked and spoke quickly, although words were few and far between with her. Mercedes was prudent with money, prudent with conversation, and prudent about changing her ways. Although she had quietly learned Spanish early on, she stubbornly refused to speak it, even until her death at 102.

Jamile, Mercedes' daughter and my great-grandmother, was strong and determined. Ever resourceful, she had made contacts with other immigrants in Colombia and had set up a potential business even before arriving. She had found a wholesaler of shoes and textiles and was prepared to open a store if their capital allowed. She was soon speaking the language of her new land with a marked Arabic accent while still carrying on Lebanese traditions at home.

As the women began their Colombian adventure, young Nayibe's eyes could barely keep up with the lush green beauty around her. Her fears of the unknown were quickly put to rest as she looked around and saw that the people of this new land were dressed differently but did not look so strange after all, for not unlike people who imagine the United States to be full of cowboys, Nayibe had imagined the inhabitants of Colombia all to be Indians. The melodious sounds of Spanish were not completely unfamiliar either, since in her homeland, many spoke French, another Romance language. Nayibe had a thirst for life and was already growing into the woman I would hear about in my mom's stories.

As soon as they arrived in Cali, Jamile registered Nayibe for school, and she began to learn Spanish. In a few days, both she and her mother Jamile were defending themselves in the new language. With the money that Mercedes had brought, they achieved their goal of opening a store in Cali much like the one they had had back home. Jamile ran the store and Mercedes ran the household. They found they even had enough to purchase their own home in a good neighborhood in Cali. They learned as they went, relied on instinct, and lived out the lessons my mom would tirelessly repeat to me:

"There is never room for failure if you have given it a good and earnest try."

"Even if you don't reach your goal, you only fail if you have not tried."

"Simply by trying you have already achieved the most important part."

My *abuela* Nayibe continued her studies but only finished through junior high. Then she went to work full-time at the family store. By this time she had blossomed into an elegant and beautiful young woman. She was confident and she was strong. Her attire was always impeccable, and she carried herself with an air of pride, yet she was always quick with a smile. She was quite a conversationalist and loved to visit the homes of others after work to discuss different issues of the day, both serious and gossipy.

Up to this point, the new life in Colombia had been good to Mercedes, Jamile, and Nayibe. Their home eventually became something of a halfway house for newly arrived Lebanese immigrants, whom they would help to get on their feet. Charity flowed in their blood as much as capitalism, and the refugees would leave forever grateful to these three interesting and complicated women.

During her work at the family store my *abuela* Nayibe met her future husband, Alvaro, a handsome man who was selling merchandise door-to-door. Nayibe's mother, Jamile, had a weakness for good-looking young men—if he was handsome, then he was perfect for her daughter. My grandfather Alvaro was just that. Well-dressed, dapper, and a gentleman, he not only quickly swept Nayibe off her feet, but he also gained swift approval from his soon-to-be mother-in-law, Jamile, and the ultimate family matriarch, Mercedes.

However, not all was what it seemed. Alvaro was truly a good man with a heart of gold, but he had no head for finance. After the wedding, the women allowed him too much access to the family business, and in less than one year they were financially ruined. He had several weaknesses. One was drinking; the other was giving away merchandise to anyone claiming he could not pay for it. This did not sit well with his tightfisted in-laws. Charity was one thing, but going out of business was another. But Alvaro was generous beyond reason and funny, funny, funny! Years later, my grandfather would sit himself down in our tiny little plastic pool, leaving hardly any room for the kids, making us giggle for hours. Or he'd have me in stitches on the floor with a silly gag that he did with a rubber chicken, a tiny ukulele, and a Groucho Marx mustache. He had a way of charming his way into your heart.

After his death, we found out that Alvaro had helped many indigent families in Cali. Quietly, without telling another soul, he would buy shoes for other parents' children and put food on the tables of those he met who were in need. However, even though he left the women of the family high and dry, he was never asked to leave, as money did not rule over love, even to the women who carried cash close to their hearts. They accepted him with all of his shortcomings, and in the end, Alvaro would prove the depth of his love for Nayibe beyond any doubt.

In the meantime, to make ends meet, Jamile and Nayibe somehow found the means to take on a little storefront. They sewed simple dresses and made rag dolls, and as often as they sold them for pesos, they would barter them for fruit and food.

Even though Alvaro's wandering eye made the marriage between him and Nayibe difficult from the beginning, their union produced seven children—five girls and two boys. My *tia* America was Nayibe's firstborn. My mom was the middle child. After my mom, Nayibe and Alvaro waited seven years before having the last three, creating a younger group of children that the four older children would ultimately have to raise.

As the next generation was born, the family was struggling financially. Alvaro was rarely home; he was usually out trying to stir up some business and deal with his own demons. Once again, it was a woman's world. Mercedes would use the handmade rag dolls to create a fantasy world in the kitchen patio for her great-grandchildren. Nayibe became the strong one now. Now that she was responsible for seven young lives, she lost a bit of her easy attitude. Although she ran a strict household, as the older children became teenagers, her home became a social center. Having so many daughters, five in all, she preferred to have their suitors come to her house rather than have her girls go out, even with an ever-present chaperone.

On weekends, the house would have music and food and drink, even if it had to be brought by the suitors themselves. The boys knew the rules and learned how to play the game as well. The secret was for them to place some candy in their coat pockets and pretend not to notice as Mercedes would slyly pickpocket it, to her stomach's delight. And every once in a while, one of the young suitors—my father, Gregorio, included—would rent a small bus, and as many as could fit would drive to a river valley out in the country for a day's retreat. Nayibe would go along under the guise of chaperone, but she really just enjoyed the camaraderie.

Piecing the story of their lives together, I find that both a strong work ethic and altruism flow through the generations; the women worked hard but they gave generously. And there was always a love of people and family: homes were always open, food was always served even when the coffers were not so full, and they used their creative resources to make all feel welcome. Later on, although my more contemplative nature probably kept my homes a bit quieter than theirs were, I, too, found hard work and charity to be a reliable formula for success.

As I contemplate my mother's upbringing in Nayibe's household and the stories of the women before her, I can see where much of my mom's personality comes from. But one event in particular would change the course of our family history forever: at the age of forty-one, when Nayibe's oldest daughter, America, was nineteen and her youngest son was only four, my mother's mother suddenly felt terribly ill. It was 1957.

Chapter 4

A TRADITION OF SILENCE

*T*here was only one doctor in Cali who would attend to women with "lumps" in their chest. Although he told Nayibe, Alvaro, and their oldest daughter, America, that Nayibe had cancer, no one used that word again once they returned home. From that point forth she was suffering from "tumors," and it was not to be discussed.

She would get better.

It could be no other way.

No one was to upset her and no one was to cry in front of her. The tradition of cancer began here, but this is also where a tradition of silence started to take hold of my family.

Our family was not unusually private. But the things that shamed my family into silence are the same things that have caused Hispanic women to die from breast cancer at a rate greater than that of their Anglo counterparts. In my life, I have vowed to break this silence and shine light on the cultural barriers, which were and are too plentiful: Women being afraid to be diagnosed, women fearing their husbands will leave them if they lose their breasts. Women believing that God will fix the problem, women believing it will go away if they leave it alone. Women believing they can't afford the cure or will die anyway, so why bother? Husbands refusing to allow their wives' or daughters' breasts to be examined by another man, even a physician. Wives believing that taking care of the problem would be putting their own care before the care of their family, which would go against every value they had been taught.

Ignorance is what keeps many of us in fear and denial. This is what I have been fighting so hard to change.

Like too many Latina women even today, my grandmother found out too late, and the doctor in Cali could not offer her much hope or many options. Somehow, with the help of their eldest child, America, who was working at an accounting office, they collected the funds to go to Bogotá, the capital of Colombia. At the Instituto de Nacional Cancerología, they sought help from the only place in the entire country that actually treated women with "tumors."

They quickly operated on my *abuela* and performed a hideous radical mastectomy, removing her left breast. Fortunately, this surgical procedure has long since been improved, but not until after millions of women were amputated and grossly disfigured. Nayibe had no forewarning about the procedure—only when she woke up did she find out that her breast had been removed. As follow-up to the surgery, they burned her skin with yet unrefined levels of radiation. Even in her skin's raw state they continued the radiation. As I am living proof, this too has evolved significantly, and today's highly advanced treatments are now targeted, quick, and effective. Unfortunately, no one questioned the medical team, nor did they ask specifics about the surgery or how the radiation would affect her. My grandparents were told this had to be done and they followed doctors' orders. That was just how it was done back then.

Abuela never came to terms with the mutilation of her body. There were no support groups, no therapy, no one to talk to, no one to emulate. She was alone. And yet her illness and these barbaric attempts at treatment would not dominate her.

After this trauma, Nayibe and Alvaro returned home. She arrived less than the woman she was when she left, not just physically but spiritually. Despite being in great pain, she managed to put on a wide smile and greet her children upon arrival. But all the power of her strong will could not contain the cancer that had already gotten the upper hand over her body. Nayibe quickly continued to fall deeper and deeper into the strong grip of the breast cancer monster.

Throughout her decline, she insisted on putting on a brave face for her children and her family. Amazingly, Nayibe applied makeup and styled her beautiful gray-streaked hair every day. It was superficial and senseless, maybe, but as a woman with breast cancer now, I understand. At least she would not look like she felt. Sometimes presenting a strong facade helps fortify what is crumbling inside.

Admirably, she even made a makeshift prosthetic out of cloth to fill out her bra. Life would go on, but soon, about seventeen months after the trip to Bogotá, she became bedridden. The disease would ultimately overtake the stubbornness of her will.

Her mother, Jamile, cared for Nayibe during the day, and then Stella, another of my aunts, would take care of her at night. America and Stella, Nayibe's first- and second-born children, barely out of their teens, were now financially responsible for the household, as Alvaro still proved unable to be a reliable breadwinner. The constant ebb and flow of suitors and other visitors who normally frequented the house, especially on weekends, trickled down to a mere few, and now, after entering, they knew they could not climb the stairs to the second floor where Nayibe lay. The second floor was for no one but the family, access governed by an unspoken rule that the reality of what was happening there was not to be shared with others.

The cancer continued to spread quickly throughout Nayibe's body. Alvaro, Jamile, Mercedes, and the oldest children became even more desperate when science stopped offering them any hope whatsoever. Nayibe had been the financial glue of the family, and her surgery had been expensive. As a result, the family was financially indebted beyond recovery. Yet anything and everything would be done to give her hope and a chance to get better.

During the most helpless times, a desperate mind often finds reason in the most implausible places. Alvaro and some of his friends heard that the blood of a rooster had cured some other women with "tumors" just like Nayibe's. The old wives' tale held that the strange blood would stimulate the immune system and fight off the cancer. The men went around the city and countryside and finally stumbled upon a doctor who would assist them with the transfusions. They asked everyone they knew to donate rooster blood so that Nayibe could get better. But as with so many women who suffered from breast cancer at that time and in that country, eventually the pain was just too severe and the illness was all people could see when they looked at her wasting body.

Finally, with pain that ran deep into the center of his heart, Alvaro approached his mother-in-law, Jamile, to discuss keeping Nayibe out of so much pain. The result would be a steady dose of morphine, most of which had to be acquired underground through a black market. At the time, palliative care was unheard of and high levels of morphine for the terminally ill were illegal. No matter, everyone wanted to help, and Alvaro's friends would come to the house with morphine hidden in their overcoat pockets.

On June 29, 1959, a little less than two years after that first visit to the doctor, Nayibe died in her sleep at the age of forty-three. She left behind seven children, the youngest of whom was six years old. Although Alvaro had had times of absence, and although he hadn't been able to properly provide for his family, in the end, the depth of his love was apparent. Alvaro would never recover from the loss, and from that moment forward Jamile would wear only black. Her daughter's death threw her into a lifetime of mourning.

Nayibe's eldest, my *tia* America, was twenty-one at the time, and my mom, Yamila, was sixteen. The death of my grandmother affected my mom terribly. She was immediately forced to drop out of school and help raise her two younger sisters and her baby brother. Furthermore, as I would later find out myself, you never truly recover from watching your mother waste away from cancer. The intense burning may subside, but it stays with you and subconsciously lurks beneath many of your decisions and life choices.

As I heard this story from my mom years ago and as I hear my aunts tell it to me now, one striking detail still rings through. They all made a point of telling me that up until her body and mind were no longer connected, Nayibe never once complained of pain or pitied her situation. Undoubtedly she suffered. She endured unimaginable pain. But like so many women in my family, she did so behind the veil of hope-filled eyes. She lived and died true to the meaning of her Arabic name: Nayibe, noble and elegant.

Pain is a reality I have had to deal with for years. I know with certainty that I've inherited a trait that helps me manage pain beyond the average person's threshold. As I learned about the life of Nayibe, and as you will read about my *tia* America and my mom, we have all found a way to strengthen our minds relative to the weakening of our bodies. There is no martyrdom here. I believe this ability stems from a physiological mutation involving nerve signals to the brain that we manage to override by our own power of mind. We work through it, we push it away, we pray for the strength to endure it without letting it break down the only thing we can count on—hope.

Although Nayibe was told it was in vain, she fought valiantly against the cancer that was permeating her every cell. She embraced her reality as soon as it became clear to her. She acknowledged her mortality and simply let it be. My aunts believed that as a woman, she made peace with her death, although I used to wonder how she reconciled with leaving her children behind. Later on, my own mother would resolve that question for me.

Chapter 5

A STRUGGLE TO SURVIVE, A SURPLUS OF LOVE

*I*n Colombia, as in so many other Latin American countries, a person's potential is often decided at birth. If you come from a prominent family with a well-known last name, chances are you will attend one of the best schools, start a promising career, and, of course, marry someone who also comes from a "good" family. Back in the 1960s the idea of someone working their way up and improving their destiny in Colombia was still a vague concept. Had my mother and father stayed there, I strongly doubt I would have become the person I am today. I am an example of the American Dream, and as much as I honor my Colombian roots and have strived to live biculturally, the state of mind instilled in me—that everything was possible and nothing was off limits—was clearly a value acquired from living in the United States.

My mom's name, Yamila, is a Colombian version of her grandmother's name, the Persian *Jamile*, which she would later symbolically change to the more American "Jamie." Yamila had always been very attached to her mother and father (Nayibe and Alvaro), her six siblings, and her grandmother and great-grandmother (Jamile and Mercedes). But losing her mom pushed her into adulthood at an early age and further strengthened her reliance on her remaining family, especially her older sisters, Stella and America.

Whereas my mom was born into a "good" family that had hit rough economic times, my father, Gregorio, was born to a mother who had settled in Cali after walking from her little native town hundreds of miles away. He never met his father and, from the age of six, was pulled out of school to work. Unlike my mother, who was surrounded by familial support, he became distanced from his mother and his brother and practically had to raise himself. Fortunately, he had a good head on his shoulders, and he taught himself how to survive and excel.

To see where he ended up is worthy of respect. From these humble beginnings and low expectations, to have led his family as well as he did is inspiring in its own way. But ours is a different bond. Because of what he never knew growing up, he never knew what to give his own family in the way of open communication and tenderness. He shows his love in quiet ways, but unlike the physical affection I was able to express with my mom, there is a gauzy wall between me and my father that keeps us farther apart.

It was my music that brought my dad and me together. When I was five, my father did not hesitate to get me a guitar after he saw my eyes light up as I watched my uncle play during a family gathering. He quietly and faithfully supported my dream of becoming an artist. Even so, I waited in vain for him to became the parent that my mother was, but I finally learned that people can only be who they are. She was one way and he is another; that is the way it is. But the more I learned about where he came from, that he was distanced from his siblings, that through sheer sweat and determination he secured basic but decent jobs, and that he dreamed of a life in another land, the easier it was to understand him and to accept the limitations of our relationship.

My mom and dad were married in 1960, less than two years after my *abuela* Nayibe died. My mom was eighteen. During my parents' engagement, my father told my mother of his desire to leave Colombia. He was starry-eyed in his belief that in America he could forge a better life for them and especially for the family they would one day start. Later on she told me that she had hesitated to agree to his plan, but ultimately she left the decision in his hands. Seven years later she found herself experiencing a snowy, blistering cold winter in a place called New Jersey. Like her mother before her, she had made an exodus from her homeland, hoping for a better life. But unlike her mother, she was leaving behind her family. She often said that deciding to leave her siblings was one of the hardest things she ever did, but the fact that she did so is testament to the way my father had swept her off her feet.

Once in the States, she found a shocking, different life. Simply to pay rent on a tiny apartment, to put food on the table, and to take care of the basics of his young family, my dad had to work two and even three jobs at a time.

This was in the late 1960s and unlike today, there was not a large Hispanic community in northern New Jersey. My mom was accustomed to being surrounded by family and friends, and this isolated existence hit her quite hard. Little by little, however, she met other people and started to learn the language, but the culture shock was abrupt and affected her deeply. Not until many years later would she be able to spread the wings of her personality that had been clipped by the loss of her mother and the move to a strange new homeland.

I was born in New Jersey in 1969, but when I was still in diapers, my parents decided to return to Colombia. My mom wanted to be near her sisters at this time in her life, and we stayed long enough for me to start kindergarten there.

She would walk me to school every day. You could say she was a bit overprotective, but we were a team, and I was her little girl.

My earliest memories are filled with joy and love. My aunts, uncles, and cousins were always around, and in this big extended family, I had a clear sense that I belonged. The soundtrack of my youth was filled with homemade music and raucous laughter, all bound together by food and by the bloodline we shared.

Soon after that, my father heard his calling again, and we packed our bags once more. This time we would stay in New Jersey for good. In order to make it work this time, my parents worked hard to fully embrace the American experience. They worked on their English, studied American history, and with bright eyes and new clothes became U.S. citizens. Our life was set to continue, but it would be in sharp contrast to the life we had left behind.

Throughout my childhood, both my parents worked extremely hard. We spent time with my father mostly on Sundays, as he would work overtime whenever he could. We barely got by, even with all their work. Fortunately, my mom was creative. When there was no money for clothes, she would sew my dresses from remnants she would find on sale at the local fabric store. At the neighborhood supermarket, where she and my father used a secret whistle to call back and forth to each other, they would step aside at the checkout counter to calculate exactly what they could purchase, making sure the coupons were correct and then returning items to the shelves until what we had in our cart was back under the limit. We could not afford a vacation, but my parents took us on inexpensive day trips to beaches and museums that not only enriched our lives but helped us forget about what we did not have. If I said I was bored, my mom, as in the stories I would hear about my great-great-grandmother Mercedes, would entertain me by inventing games like sitting face-to-face to see who could make the other laugh first, or acting out made-up stories while she did housework.

We never had extras, nor did we have many comforts, but what we did have was a surplus of love. Meals were eaten as a family, laughter was ever-present, and letters flowed freely between my mom and her sisters back in Colombia. My mother, just like her mother, loved to have people in her home. Our door would always be open, and no event could go by without some sort of celebration. She made homemade piñatas, baked beautiful birthday cakes, and put together amazing homemade party favors. However humble our situation might have been, she did her best to ensure that everyone felt welcome, making up for what we lacked in fancy food and a big home with sheer charisma and a loving disposition.

Somehow, she made it work. She took so much pride in putting up a positive front that we never looked as if we were struggling. Every day she would dress me up and fuss over my hair, which she would wash and untangle at night and place in pigtails or braids in the morning. Unfortunately for my adolescent social life, she would not allow me to change this hairstyle until I was a freshman in high school.

I look back at this now and can only wonder. My parents found a way around every struggle. How did they do it? I can only imagine what their conversations were like behind closed doors. Now, every dollar I earn I respect. To this day, I find it hard to splurge. I spend only what I have. I am so aware of what it feels like to have no financial security that I never want to go back there again. A couple of years ago I finally built my dream house, and I thank my parents every time I walk in the front door. It is incomprehensibly beautiful to me, but its appeal comes not from indulgence and grandeur, but from careful planning, the crafts-manship of special hands, and the way it honors nature's beauty and my Colombian roots. Everything my mother taught me about hard work, charity and generosity, and prudence and humility has brought me to this place where I can afford to live out my dreams and close my eyes every night knowing that I have arrived here without harming anyone and, I hope, by doing plenty of good along the way. I am also grateful to my father for risking it all for his family. By moving us so far away, he showed me the importance of taking risks in the hope of achieving something greater for ourselves and those around us. By somehow find-ing the time to earn a GED and a college degree while working full-time, he taught me tenacity. Ultimately, the brick and mortar of my life's successes are built from my parents' sweat and sacrifices.

My spare childhood might have prompted me to earn well and save carefully, but it is the values of my upbringing that have kept me from losing focus on what truly matters. If the financial demands of my health care ever outstrip my resources, I know I could go back to living in that tiny little apartment in North Jersey if I had to. Practical things would change, but my essence would still be the same.

Once I was in elementary school full-time, my mom began work-ing a variety of hard manual-labor jobs. At first she worked in an underwear factory, sewing the final lace trim on the undergarments. In Colombia, my mom would never have done the kind of work she did here in the United States. In that environment, which is more con-scious of social status, these jobs would have been beneath her, but she put her pride aside and did what she had to in order to help the family. Along the way, this taught me a great lesson. I've had many opportunities to be a starving musician, playing low-paying gigs or waiting for royalty checks for songs. But her hard work, the sweat of the women before me, and my Lebanese heritage have combined to give me a nose for finding business opportunities. Instead of shunning endorsements, for example, I chose to embrace corporate America, joining hands with quality products I believe in, in exchange for help in getting my message out about awareness and early detection of breast cancer. My ability to see clearly that I should do whatever it takes came from my mom.

The underwear factory where my mom worked was right across the street from where we lived. She worked there for a few years and forged some beautiful friendships. During that time I watched my mom become more vocal, and I loved it when she would invite some of her coworkers over after their shift. They would sit around the kitchen table and drink coffee and snack and just talk. I would linger around them, hoping she would ask me to play them a song. Then I would do the usual—act shy at first, then give in and get my guitar. I was involved in after-school activities like soccer and music, and that gave her a little more time for herself as I got older.

Nevertheless, just like her mom and her mom's mom before her, though they succeeded to a certain extent in acclimating to their new home country, some habits were just too hard to break. My lunch box never featured peanut butter and jelly. I would have to explain to curious onlookers why my rice was yellow and what *arepas* and *empanadas* were. Through language, food, and holiday traditions, my mom fought to hold onto the customs that linked her to both her Lebanese and her Colombian cultures. New Year's Eves were always fun in our house. We would eat the traditional grapes, pour the glass of water out the window, and run around in each room in the apartment with an empty suitcase to bring on lots of travel (I think she made this one up to keep us entertained!), and she would break an egg into water and tell us our future. She would make tabouli and kibbe one weekend, and the next we would have *sancocho de gallina*.

As a child, I had a tendency to be a bit of a loner. I was an excellent, disciplined student with not an ounce of rebellion in me. When I came home from school, I would rush to do my homework, and then I would sit for hours practicing the violin and playing my guitar and singing. I rarely had friends over, as I found more comfort and enjoyment in playing my music and being with my mom. I was terribly attached to her. Even back then, something inside of me pushed me not to stop until I had completed a task, never to give up, and to believe that nothing was out of reach.

In that little New Jersey apartment in Bergenfield, my mom loved to hear me practice, and she would often ask me to come and play in the kitchen while she prepared dinner or in the living room as she ironed my dad's shirts. This time was so important for me. Both my parents were very supportive of my musical talents and aspirations, but it was these private concerts that inspired me to practice hour after hour, day after day.

Although she could not even carry a tune whistling and it was actually painful to hear her sing, my mother loved music. On the sly I would ask my dad to teach me the lyrics of Colombian songs just so I could surprise her with a little touch of home during my next serenade. Much of who I am today was born during those afternoons. My mother urged me to never be afraid to take a chance. She encouraged me to go against the wind if my convictions were strong enough. She instilled in me a sense of self-worth and self-esteem based solely on values and not measured against outside standards or opinions.

I learned so much from my mother. As with the women before her, charity ran deep in her blood. We had to stretch our groceries like rations, but there was always enough for an extra person to join us. We lived in cramped quarters, but our home was always open. Many times, I remember going out with her to run an errand and watching her give away what little she had in her wallet to people who seemed like they needed it more. Once, on our way to put a payment down for something she had placed on layaway, I clearly remember having to return home because she had found another soul to nurture. She taught me that if someone truly needed money, you had to give him what you had, and if you lived like that, you would never run into hard times—whatever you gave would somehow be replenished, because that is just how the balance in life works. Sure enough, when times got really rough, someone would step forward to help us, our luck would turn around, and we would always bounce back, and from that my mother's own innate sense of karma was passed along to me.

Just before I began high school, we moved to Point Pleasant, another town in New Jersey, right on the Atlantic Ocean. Things had gotten rough in our Bergenfield neighborhood, and it had become hard for me at school. I kept it from my parents until one day my mom caught me out of breath as I was walking up the stairs to our apartment. It didn't take much to figure out that I was a walking target for bullies. I wore clothes that were clean but a bit out of style, my hair was up in pigtails (even in middle school), I carried my violin to school every day, and I loved to sit in the front row of my classes, do extra homework, and, yes, be the teacher's pet. Fortunately, I had a best friend, Tanya, a track runner, who taught me that I could outrun this bunch of kids who had taken a liking to harassing me—violin and heavy book bag and all!

When my parents found out what was going on, it pushed them over the edge. The neighborhood had changed, and they were uncomfortable staying. But there was the problem of money. Where would we go, and how would we afford it? A guardian angel stepped in, and the balance of life tipped our way again. Through a friend of a friend, my parents heard of a house that needed to be sold. The price was fair enough so that we could afford the monthly payments, but we did not have the money for the down payment. My *tia* America's business was doing well, and she came forward and gave us the money. After fifteen years in this country, my parents took a major step toward achieving the American Dream by buying their first home.

In this new oceanside town, my mom took a new job. She worked as a cleaning lady at a motel that was within walking distance of our new home. My mom never learned how to drive, so the proximity of her job to our house was important for her continued independence. The job was hard, hard work. She would come home dead tired, her knees and back sore from bending and lifting all day, her hands worn from the cleaning supplies. At this point I was in high school, and she was confiding in me more and more. She would complain about how dirty some people were and how so few of them would leave any tip for the housekeeping department. To this day when I travel, I make a point of saying hello to the housekeeping staff and of saying thank you when they clean my room, and I always leave them a little something when I check out. Most people don't even notice the housekeeper, but I see my mother in their eyes and I always wonder what the family is like that is dependent on that paycheck. I always wonder what hidden dreams these women have set aside in order to make ends meet.

My mom also did babysitting and other miscellaneous jobs. In the end, not only did she help the family's bottom line, but these jobs helped her define her identity beyond being a wife and a mother. She was able to have her own money and control her own finances. She was also able to meet more people and form a circle of friends who would serve as a surrogate extended family for her.

When I was in high school, my mother's English improved, and she became more outspoken and more like the young woman she had been in her homeland. Every once and a while, my *tias* would come and visit, and a handful of times, when there was a special airfare or when my dad could get a loan against future earnings, my mom and I would spend our summer vacation in Cali with the rest of her family.

When I was in high school, it dawned on me that I not only had to continue to be an overachiever, but I had to raise it up a notch. It was clear that my parents would not be able to afford to pay my college tuition, and I was determined not to be left behind or swallowed up by thousands of dollars of student loan debt. So I set up a meeting with a guidance counselor my first year and asked her what I needed to do. By the time I graduated, I was valedictorian, president of the student council, a member of the National Honor Society, captain of the field hockey team, a member of the all-county chorus, and then some. I did everything to excel, took every advanced placement class possible, and then applied to every scholarship that I could possibly qualify for. I wanted a first-class education. That is what my parents had sacrificed so hard for, and I was not going to let anything get in my way.

The year I went off to college, my mom was arguing with her doctor about some tests. She insisted that they redo a mammogram because something inside of her did not feel quite right. Finally, they redid the test, and in a few brief minutes in a cold room in a doctor's office, life as we knew it changed forever.

Crossroads

Jamie said my body's tired
I've got to get some rest
I've been pacing around for hours
Trying to understand this fate

Step by step
And around I go, in and out of my memories

A flashback here,
A vision there,
I never quite felt so free

Strange how some moments have just faded
Strange how some feelings just aren't there

And I'm standing at the crossroads of this world
That waits for me
It lures me with caresses like a feather on my cheek
Soothing me to sleep

And all the restlessness that consumed me has disappeared
And all my yearnings to fight it have gone with my last tear

I throw my life into the hands of a force I cannot see
I pull away from what I know and unite with what I believe in

Strange how some moments have just faded
Strange how some feelings just aren't there

(continued)

31

Crossroads (continued)

And I'm standing at the crossroads of this world
That waits for me
It lures me with caresses like a feather on my cheek
Soothing me to sleep

Though I've loved you all
I know I've earned my turn
To think of me and only me

Here's to all we've known
To the cross that we have borne
Something is coming
To set me free . . .

And I'm standing at the crossroads of this world
That waits for me
It lures me with caresses like a feather on my cheek

Chapter 6

MOTHER AND DAUGHTER

I went to Douglass College at Rutgers University. Had it not been for the generosity of so many people and organizations, I would never have made it through like I did. I went to the college of my choice on a full academic scholarship and ended my four-year university studies with two thousand dollars left over with which to get a head start in life. Douglass was a prestigious women's college with a pastoral campus and an amazing liberal arts program. Although I had chosen to live on campus, the university was only about an hour's drive from home. That short hop on the Garden State Parkway would become my salvation for the next four years.

"There is a large tumor in the left breast, and there also seems to be activity in her lymph nodes under her left arm." So began the conversation with my mom's new oncologist.

I had come home from school to go with her to the appointment. Her family physician had found the lump during an examination and had sent her to get a mammogram, and the results of the mammogram called for a follow-up with an oncologist. In a short span of time, she found out she would need to have her left breast removed and undergo heavy rounds of chemotherapy. It was 1987, and my mom was forty-six years old, only five years older than her mother had been when she faced a similar diagnosis.

In his office she sat speechless and emotionless. It was like a punch to the stomach, and we both had had the air knocked out of us. My mom was so strong, so active. Years before, she had had a bout with thyroid cancer, but that was now under control and she hardly even got colds. Here we were listening to the most absurd, frightening proclamation from a man we had just met. Like my mom, I could barely muster a word. I watched her go completely blank. I told him we needed time to take it all in and that we would call him later with questions.

Leaving the oncologist's office, we could hardly look at each other, and as she seemed to turn inward, I worried she might never break her silence. But then we were in the car, with the doors and windows closed.

"Your father," was the first thing she said. Then she began to sob.

"We're going to get through it, *mami*, don't worry. You are going to beat this thing," I urged her, while swallowing back my own tears of fear and confusion.

She later told me that a million thoughts raced through her head and blocked out my voice, the main one being the memory of her own mother, Nayibe, and her painful and ultimately losing battle with breast cancer. My mom had never met a woman who had survived breast cancer, and this was all she knew: breast cancer equals suffering equals dying. She had been by her mother's side and saw not only the devastating toll that cancer took on her body but also the numbing effect it had on those around her.

I had never seen my mom like this before. She was frail and lost. My role in our relationship had just changed as well. Her arms had always been my source of comfort, but now I had to grow up fast, and fast was not fast enough. She did not express to me what she was feeling. Inside of her something just simply shut down. I was only eighteen and struggling to figure out what to say and do, but I fell short. She needed me now, and I had no idea what she was going through or how to help her get through this. I had never known a breast cancer survivor either, and I did not have anyone to ask for guidance. All I knew was what my mom had gone through taking care of her mother. I was still a teenager living on my own for the first time and doing the things that one does when first tasting liberty. I wanted to be carefree, but I could not dare to be. I was struggling to be a good daughter, while fighting off the natural urge to be self-absorbed. At that age, I was unable to understand the changing dynamics in her relationship with her husband, in her own identity, in her faith, and in her life.

I split my time between college and home. I know I could have done more, but life taught me the needed skills a bit too late. Seeing and experiencing a lot of the same changes in my own body fifteen and twenty years later, I can only now begin to understand how alone and isolated she must have felt.

But eventually, long after the initial shock of her diagnosis, I witnessed an incredible change in my mom. Somehow, a remarkable transformation took place inside the soul of this woman. Arriving home from school one weekend, I was greeted by a person who had seen her path and decided she should get on it and ride. Her eyes were bright, her posture erect and proud. She used positive language to explain her situation. Something had clicked on inside of her, and she was ready to fight. She urged me to help her research her disease so she could understand it better. And she convinced herself that it was a godsend that she was in the United States, because if she was going to have a fighting chance, it would be with the help of the doctors of this country. There had been enough crying. It was time to take the upper hand.

What followed was difficult. She had a mastectomy of her left breast and many rounds of chemotherapy. Back in 1987 there were not as many drugs available to combat the side effects, and the treatment protocols were different and more limited. Fortunately, we have advanced greatly since then, but my mom suffered a lot. The antinausea medicine did nothing for her, and it seemed as if she was always sick. She cried when her hair fell out, she cried when she felt ill. But those things eventually subsided. Hair does eventually grow back and the chemo does eventually work its way out of your system.

My most painful memory is of helping her shower after her mastectomy. I had never seen "that" before, and I did all I could not to react to the sight of her concave, scar-lined chest. My mom was struggling with seeing her new body for the first time without the bandages. Again, she worried about my father.

After getting her into her clothes, we sat on her bed and talked.

"*No me siento como una mujer,*" she would mumble. "I do not feel like a woman." All I could do was hug her gently, since I did not have the words to alleviate her fears and insecurities.

Notwithstanding all the physical pain and emotional insecurities, after every breakdown, she would rise up even stronger. She sculpted a model of behavior that I would follow years later. Following this episode, my mom decided she wanted to eat better. She went off to a self-empowering retreat filled with meditation and organic foods. She read voraciously and embraced the idea that one must make the best out of what one has. She bought a wooden plaque of the well-known prayer "God grant me the serenity to accept the things I cannot change, the courage to change the things I can, and the wisdom to know the difference." She read it aloud daily, and it now hangs in my home as a testament to the power of its words.

But as it happened with her mom, no amount of positive thought or good intentions could keep her body from falling deeper into the grips of the disease. It was terrifying to watch the cancer move. It was equally terrifying to watch the effects of the treatments and impossible to accept all of their limitations. But it was awe-inspiring to watch her slowly learn to accept her reality.

Both of her arms were swollen by then. She had lymphedema. Often, when a woman has a mastectomy and the lymph nodes under her arms are removed, her lymphatic system, which provides purification and drainage for the body, becomes compromised. Any trauma like a burn or an infection can cause the lymphatic system to overload and clog and therefore cause disfiguring swelling. Both of my mom's arms had a mild but painful case of this swelling. Unfortunately, I now know what this feels like—it feels like your limbs belong to a dead man. Both arms were affected, because by this point in her disease her right breast had also been removed. Today we know that manual massages can relieve the buildup of fluid, and there are compression bandages and sleeves to help. Now we know that if caught early enough, lymphedema can be reversed. But when my mom was sick in the late 1980s, providing relief from lymphedema didn't seem to be a priority for her doctors.

My mother never chose to undergo surgical reconstruction of her breasts. Actually, she was never able to seriously consider it since in her case, every waking moment was spent fighting the disease, and she never had a chance to catch her breath between treatments. After a while, her mastectomy scars became a badge of courage for her. I vividly remember the last trip she took to Colombia to see her siblings, when she just opened up her blouse and showed her scarred and burned chest to her sisters. Choosing just to be herself, she hadn't even packed her bra prosthetic. What a remarkable transformation from that afternoon when I helped her shower. I can only wonder how much of it was sheer poker face and how much was genuine acceptance. I know she still cried herself to sleep sometimes, and only now can I begin to piece it together. Watching her embrace the trauma to her body and witnessing her reunion with her own femininity helped me find myself when I thought that my own essence had also been amputated.

In the midst of the pain, the operations, the constant chemotherapy, radiation, and all of the side effects, she somehow found a way to live.

The company my father worked for was moving its office from New York to south Florida, and my father was being transferred as well. I had just graduated from college and was working as a flight attendant based out of New York. Although I had a degree in English literature, I was focused on earning enough money to record a demo to shop my music to a major record label. Since I spoke Spanish, I was given Latin American routes and was able to continue writing songs while listening to the music of places like Argentina, Chile, and countries in Central America. I moved with my parents to Boca Raton and commuted to New York by plane. The arrangement was right for the time.

Again, my *tia* America was there for us, giving my father the down payment so that he could buy my mom her dream home. My father was now a more educated man, working as an engineer for a company that manufactured ceramics. He was responsible with money and long ago had paid my aunt back for the down payment on our New Jersey home. But still, it wasn't common then for a Hispanic executive to rise quickly in white-collar America, and our family income was still modest. The home was nice, but by most standards it wasn't much of a dream home. It was a small, simple townhouse in a cookie-cutter development. But for my mother it was a castle! She loved that it was new. She loved the kitchen. She finally had her own bathroom with a separate shower, a big bathtub, and her own sink. There was a community pool with a clubhouse, and she could walk to the public library just down the street. She also had a little screened-in patio where she would sit for hours, surrounded by her plants, looking out onto the man-made lake and admiring all of the Florida birds that would come by. Her entire collection of clay wind chimes from Colombia hung by the main entrance, giving her a little glimpse of her past as she walked through the door every day. For a family that had been living in penny-pinching apartments that never had a view grander than a parking lot, this was the Taj Mahal.

She was so proud. Everyone she knew was invited, and as always the door was wide open. Unfortunately, she was already quite ill and was only able to enjoy her home for a little over a year, but thanks to my aunt, she was able to have that year.

The move to Florida was another step in my mother's liberation. One morning over breakfast she declared that she wanted to finally get her driver's license. I was surprised and thrilled.

"That's great! Let's do it!"

"Ay, do you think I can? *Sólo en pensarlo me siento nerviosa!*" she admitted with the excitement of a child: "Just thinking about it makes me nervous!"

That same day I went out and got her a driving manual. She studied it inside and out. I finally convinced her to start practicing. I would take her to an empty parking lot near my father's office. We would go there early in the morning—I needed to assure myself that not many cars would be around.

It was some of the best time I spent with her as an adult. We laughed and laughed. From my father I inherited the ability to stay calm in perilous situations. This was a useful skill as I sat in the passenger seat with my mom driving. She would hit the accelerator instead of the brake and vice versa. Reverse was just too much to handle! One time a local police officer came by and started asking us questions because he thought she was driving drunk. Then he put it all together and smiled and just asked us to be careful and keep the practice limited to the parking lot.

And so we kept trying, with very slow progress. Every day for weeks, we would drive up and down and in and out of the parking spaces. Once I finally convinced her to take the driving test, it took her two tries to pass the written portion. She insisted that her nerves canceled out her first try.

But the real disaster came with the road test. I waited for her in the lobby and after just a few minutes, her tester came in looking pale and shaken. My mom followed behind with a long look and a bit of her Spanish temper bubbling up. Sure enough, it had gone terribly. She got nervous and did absolutely the opposite of everything he had asked of her. Apparently, he had asked her to do the city a favor and not pursue getting a license. Well, that was that—there would be no driver's license for my mom. But as she would later joke, at least she tried, and maybe it was better this way.

Even though she filled our first year in Boca with smiles and her best efforts, she was physically exhausted. Her body was mutilated and worn. Her mind was also getting tired.

Throughout her illness my father stayed true and deeply attached to my mother, even as she went through a series of changes, both physical and emotional. At first, her faith wavered. She was angry at life and angry with God. She went through periods of frustration with her doctors, with us, and with herself. But in the end, she made amends with all of these pieces of her existence. Fortunately, she had managed to grow in the midst of all this turmoil, for what lay ahead would have been difficult for anyone to understand, much less handle.

MEMORIES

Soraya's family history from the late 1950s through 1996

*I*t was clear from the time she was in pigtails that Soraya Lamilla was a girl to watch—smart, talented, dedicated, and driven. Soraya was deeply influenced by her Colombian heritage and by the incredibly strong women in her family.

She was the granddaughter, niece, and daughter of women who died from breast cancer. And, with that legacy as her foundation, Soraya blossomed into a significant singer-songwriter who ultimately used her public status to create change on a global scale, while humbly inspiring herself and others around her to live deeply, with courage and hope.

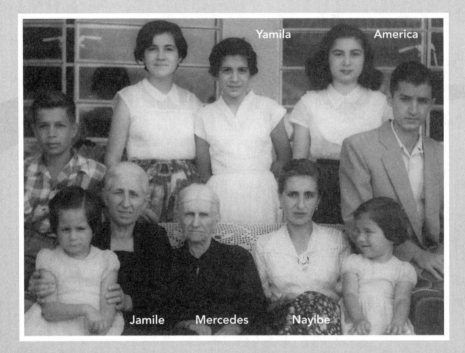

Yamila   America

Jamile   Mercedes   Nayibe

The women in Soraya's family were the foundation of her strength. In this picture, taken in the early 1950s, we see Mercedes, Soraya's great-great-grandmother, who fled from Lebanon in 1925 with daughter Jamile and granddaughter Nayibe and passed away at age 102; Jamile, Soraya's great-grandmother; Nayibe, Soraya's grandmother, who gave birth to seven children and died of breast cancer in 1959 at 43 years of age; Yamila, Soraya's mother, who died of breast cancer in 1992; and America, Soraya's aunt, who died of breast cancer in 2000.

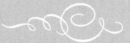

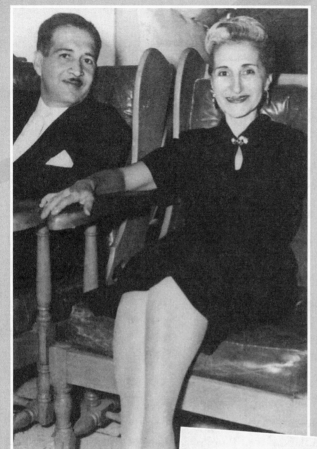

Soraya's grand-
parents, Alvaro
and Nayibe, in
1958, about one
year before
Nayibe's death.
Putting on a brave
face, Nayibe is
carefully coiffed
and fully made up.

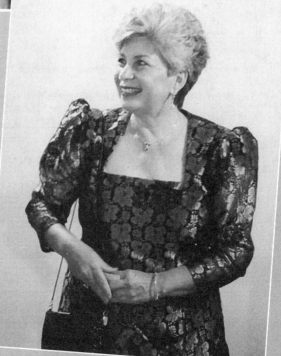

Tia America, in 1986—
the regal and business-
savvy aunt Soraya
looked up to.

oraya played the guitar right-handed, but she was a lefty. When she was a little girl, her father got her a guitar as a gift, which she had been begging for. The guitar was for a righty, but she was so thankful to have it and so anxious to play it that she willed herself the coordination she'd need to make music with it. Playing right-handed stuck for life, even after she had many chances to switch back. As part of her roots it meant something to her, and as always, she honored where she came from.

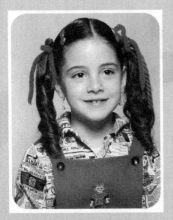

Soraya at six, already a guitar player.

oraya learned early in life that hard work paid off well. She graduated at the number-one spot in her high school class and earned a four-year scholarship to Douglass College at Rutgers University. Even as a young woman, she had an incredibly strong sense of self.

SORAYA
An excerpt from her June 1987 high school valedictorian speech

We need to understand the importance of respecting others and their thoughts and feelings. Yet at the same time we need to recognize the importance of respecting ourselves above all else. We can control who we are, what we believe in, and why we believe.

From the Point Pleasant newspaper *The Leader*, April 1987.

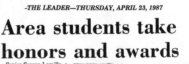

-THE LEADER—THURSDAY, APRIL 23, 1987

Area students take honors and awards

Senior Soraya Lamilla, a top student at Point Pleasant High School, epitomizes the accomplishments that come from dedication to hard work, according to Director of Pupil Personnel Sandra Zahner. Soraya is the recipient of a four-year, full-tuition scholarship to Rutgers University.

Principal Frank McLaughlin said, "Soraya has solid ability, and she has the self discipline and motivation to achieve success in whatever she does."

Soraya is also the recipient of a Garden State Distinguished Scholar Award, National Hispanic Scholars Award and another Rutgers University Scholarship.

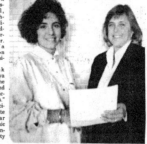

TOP STUDENT — Soraya Lamilla, left, of Point Pleasant High School, won a full four year scholarship to Rutgers University. Congratulating her is Sandra Zahner, director of Pupil Personnel at the high school.

PEGGY VAN BEVEREN
A coach, mentor, and friend

Soraya was a goalie. A great goalie. She wouldn't hesitate to dive, totally stretched out horizontally, to protect the goal. It didn't take her teammates long to appreciate her 100 percent effort on the field. Then I discovered she was an academic standout and musically gifted. This kid had it all!

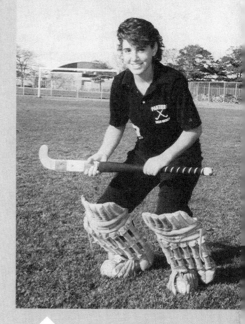

Soraya in her field hockey gear.

After one of our field hockey games Soraya introduced me to her parents. It didn't take long to see that Soraya's strong self-esteem was a product of their loving attention. As time passed, Soraya graduated valedictorian of her senior class, and I kept in touch with the Lamilla family. Lucky for me, I had been invited to a couple of family gatherings. After one dinner, Soraya asked me to listen to her sing. She got out her guitar and began to sing a song she had written. It was at that moment that I grasped the depth of passion she had for music. She gave me a tape of her playing guitar and singing. She asked for it back years later when she became famous; I sent it to her, but not before I played it one last time!

A November 1986 article in Point Pleasant's *The Leader* reported, "The talented scholar (ranked top in her senior class) and athlete registered 159 saves out of 195 shots on goal during the season. . . . While the competition finds the Borough goalie tough on the field, they should feel fortunate they do not have to meet up with her in the classroom. In addition to her top academic status, Lamilla is president of the Keyettes and Vice President of the senior class. She is also a member of the National Honor Society."

1987. Soraya during her freshman year of college with her mom, the same year Yamila was diagnosed with breast cancer.

JESSICA CUEVAS
Soraya's cousin and friend

In college, Soraya was a serious student working toward a double degree in English Lit and French philosophy because she thought majoring in music would be taking the easy way out. When it came to music as a career, the family was cautiously optimistic about where it could take her. Her mother had a huge heart and capacity to dream and believe, despite her daily practicality. I always sensed that she was afraid of the world hurting or disappointing her girl; understandably so. But still, she encouraged Soraya to go for it. Uncle Gregorio showed little emotion or excitement in general, living within that guarded cage where "if you didn't expect too much from life, you might not get let down." Still, he supported her ambitions. But no doubt, my aunt's love, attention, and excitement were essential elements in Soraya's life.

PEGGY VAN BEVEREN
A coach, mentor, and friend

In one of Soraya's calls from college I learned of her mom's diagnosis of breast cancer. At times Soraya was at school, her dad was working in the city, and her mom was going to be alone a few days a week, suffering from chemo. It was the summer and I wasn't teaching, so I volunteered to sit with her, just to be in the house if she needed something. I felt as helpless as Soraya and Gregory but was happy I could help. I remember taking Jamie for a chemo session once. Her sister Stella was visiting from Colombia and came along for the ride and moral support. Stella didn't speak English, and my Spanish is very limited, but we laughed all the way there and back until we had tears in our eyes from listening to ourselves kill each other's native languages trying to communicate. I guess it was a good way to let the tears out that we would otherwise have tried to hide that day.

SORAYA
An excerpt from an English term paper she wrote during her junior year
at Douglass, in 1989, after Yamila had had a radical mastectomy

A few days later, they removed the bandages from her chest. I had looked through medical books, preparing myself for this moment. But all of those pictures didn't help. They were cold, merely nameless body parts on the page. This was my mother. This was when I first realized what had happened to her, to my father, to our family—to me. . . .

As I lie in bed, I wonder how she feels. Does she still feel attractive, complete? Can she stand in front of a mirror—naked? Does she still believe in God?

When they cut off her breasts, it was like a part of my own destiny had been amputated. For a while, I could not bear to see them, those two scars that had brutishly replaced the supple breast that had once nurtured me. Now, time has passed, and almost a year after they told us she might die, I see the scars as beautiful saviors. When I go home from school, and hear her Spanglish, I can't help but feel extremely sentimental. She is my mom. That tough lady is mine! She has been through so much in her life, and here she is, forty-eight years up the line, rosy-cheeked, and walking every day.

I sleep less nowadays. I treat my mornings as if they were the beginnings of my last day. I treasure every moment I spend with my parents, my boyfriend, my family, my friends, and especially, the moments I spend with myself. Cancer is extremely manipulative. Its presence is at times overbearing, but if it is confronted with equal perseverance, the result can be an indescribable appreciation of life, of the ones that are loved, and of oneself.

Soraya wrote "Reason to Believe" while in college, after finding comfort in this medallion, which she found when she was desperately worried about her mother's health.

MARIA DICHIO-JOHNSON
Soraya's college friend

It was at a weekend training workshop for new resident assistants that I first met Soraya. A group of us upperclassmen were sitting around a bonfire in the middle of the woods talking about strategies for dealing with incoming freshman girls. When the training part of the evening was over, Soraya pulled out her guitar and treated us to a special song she knew in Spanish. Her talent and spirit mesmerized me. We clicked right away that weekend, and Soraya quickly became a part of a larger group of college friends, namely Jen, Claudia, Janet, and my twin sister, Giovanna. During our junior and senior years we all became very close. We ate together, partied together, and sometimes we'd

48

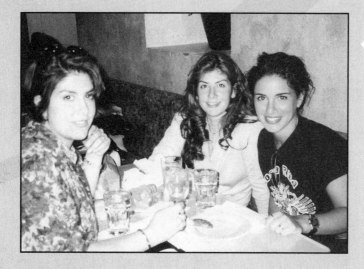

Two of Soraya's closest friends from college, twin sisters Giovanna (center) and Maria (left).

just hang out as you do in college when you should really be studying.

The bonds of our college clique have lasted since graduating in 1991, largely because of Soraya and the way her music bound us together. In our group, we had a real treat—a talented musician who would generously treat us to miniacoustic concerts throughout our time together. For those few precious moments while her voice filled the air of an otherwise stale dormitory room, her sweet vocals and beautiful soul reached out and held us suspended in another place and time.

Our group always supported Soraya through the steps she had to take to broaden her audience. One time we all trekked down to open-mike night at the coffeehouse on the Rutgers campus to see her perform to a packed audience. By then, many were familiar with her and had come out to experience the magic.

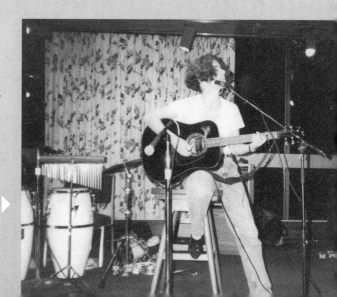

1990. Soraya performs at the coffeehouse.

In May 1991 we put together a last-minute soiree to celebrate graduation as a group with all of our families. Our plan for Operation Graduation was simple: everyone was to bring enough beer and wine for their own families, and we would open the adjoining doors to the two apartments we lived in for an impromptu double-apartment celebration. Although Soraya did not live with us, she was one of us. It was supposed to be just a quick celebratory toast and then all families would part ways to celebrate on their own. Yeah, right!!! Both apartments quickly filled up with Italians, Colombians, and enthusiastic Americans. The Latin music started pumping, and the party took off.

Before everyone said their good-byes, Soraya set up her guitar and treated us to one last concert in that same Henderson Apartment where we had shared special college memories together. Once again she ended with that special Spanish song, which everyone now knows as "Pueblito Viejo." You could see on our family's faces that they knew this moment was a snapshot into our sisterhood and the magic that Soraya brought into our group.

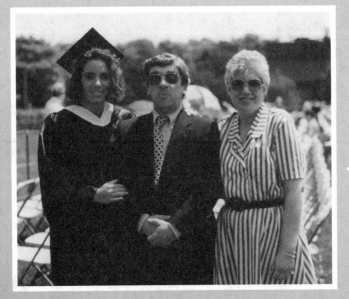

1991. Soraya at her Douglass College graduation, with proud parents Gregory and Yamila.

PEGGY VAN BEVEREN
A coach, mentor, and friend

At the end of college, Soraya had become Woman of the Year at Rutgers, her parents were moving to Florida, her mom was in remission, and she was taking a job as a flight attendant. In subsequent calls she told me she was getting a good feeling about being able to realize her passion of being a professional musician. She sent me tapes of her music along the way, and I was thrilled to get each one!

After graduation, Soraya took a job as a flight attendant for United Airlines so she could have more time to write songs and spend time with her mother in Boca Raton. Fully bilingual, the neophyte was given choice routes to South America, where the things she experienced provided musical inspiration for her songwriting.

HEIDI WEIDMAN
Soraya's United Airlines colleague and good friend

Soraya was and will always be a "fly girl"!

Back in the mid-nineties the term fly girl was being bandied around the entertainment industry, but at the time Soraya was a different type of fly girl—she was flying the friendly skies. She was originally based in New York, but when her mother's fight with cancer took a turn for the worse, she immediately put in for an emergency transfer to Miami to be closer to her family. It wasn't too long after her arrival in Miami that she was on one of my flights to South America. Let's just say it was giggles at first sight.

For Soraya, flying was only a blip on the road to her success. Always 100 percent devoted to any task, she was a great flight attendant—no surprise. A favorite of passengers because of her smile and keen sense of humor, it was a given that her fellow crew

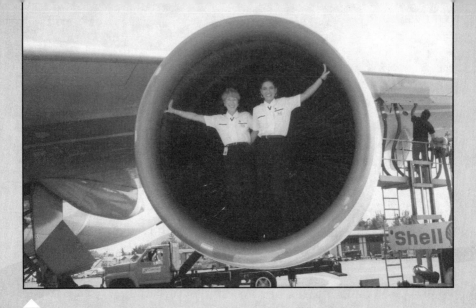

1992. Soraya and a United Airlines colleague inside a jet engine.

members fell in love with her quickly, too. On many trips to South America, she would hop on one of the hotel pianos or get a guitar that she always kept at the hotel, and entertain us with a song. Applause always followed, and an encore performance would be begged of the bubbly brunette sitting at the keyboard. She beamed from ear to ear, whether the audience was two or twenty. Can't you just picture her in the hotel lobby with a group of people mesmerized by her songs? I think the hotels even wanted to pay her; she really would gather a crowd. She loved to share the sound of music with people.

My fondest memories, however, were of the jam sessions around the pool at my apartment in Coral Gables. We were always hosting some impromptu soiree. It was poolside that we first met "Ethel," Soraya's favorite guitar. "They" would serenade us with well-known songs, and we would sing along, quite poorly as I remember. "You should be famous," we would say, and "You sound like . . ." Well, like no one really. Soraya had her own sound. Her sultry, soulful voice was captivating. Soraya had this ability to take any song and make it her very own. But when she sang her own songs, we would be incredulous that she had written such amazing words. Soraya was about sharing the gift that she had been given.

On August 21, 1992, Soraya's mom, Yamila, lost her battle with breast cancer.

PEGGY VAN BEVEREN
A coach, mentor, and friend

I remember Soraya coming to my house to tell me her mom had lost her battle with breast cancer. We cried together. She told me that she was able to be with her mom when she died and how Jamie seemed to finally be at peace. Then she told me she wrote a song about it and let me read the words. We cried some more. The song was "On Nights Like This," which later went on to become the title song of her first record.

The loss of her mother became a major theme in Soraya's writings. Here, she writes of her mom as a hero.

And if i say the words
Would all my wishes
come true
to have just one more chance
to say "i love you"
They say the world is yearning
for heroes
& here I stand being born of one

Marriott
HOTELS · RESORTS · SUITES

Reservations: 800-228-9290

*S*oraya always had a quiet confidence that she would make it in the music business. She was working hard on her craft while flying for United, but unlike other musicians who play gig after gig to attract fans and attention, Soraya was focused more on songwriting than performing. If family and friends were concerned that this quieter plan couldn't possibly lead anywhere, no one expressed it.

Then, Soraya struck up a conversation with one of her first-class passengers. He was Manolo Diaz, president of PolyGram Records. She gave him a cassette tape. It was as if Soraya had known all along exactly where she needed to put herself to meet up with her own destiny.

MANOLO DIAZ
Then president of PolyGram Records; currently oversees EMI Latin America and EMI Brazil, and serves as special advisor to Jean-François Cecillon, chairman and CEO of EMI Music International

Months later, after many more frequent-flyer miles, I was in my Coconut Grove office reading my mail, when suddenly I started to hear a song coming from far away. Even with the low intensity with which it reached my ears, it exercised a mysterious power of seduction over me. With an interesting fax half-read, I exited my office in search of this entrapping melody. It did not take long to verify that it was coming from the office of my coworker and friend, Paul Ehrlich, director of marketing for PolyGram Latin America.

"Paul, what are you listening to?" I asked him. "There is a magic to that melody."

"Well, I don't know, but it sounds beautiful," Paul answered, and then added, "I have a dozen or so demos that people have sent us, and I listen to them little by little. This is one of them. I listened to it yesterday, and I couldn't get it out of my head all

day. And look, Manolo, isn't this the cassette that you gave me
when you returned from one of your trips to Chile?"

I stood there, pensive for a while, and suddenly I remembered
and shouted: '"Yes, yes! The flight attendant from United! Let me
listen to it from the beginning." Paul and I listened—ecstatic—to
three songs by Soraya, one of them titled "Suddenly," one of the
most beautiful songs ever written.

When Manolo phoned Soraya to invite her to audition live at PolyGram Records, he introduced himself and Soraya fired back, "Ha, ha, very funny." Certain it was a prank that her friends were playing on her, she hung up on him. But soon enough, she was in the PolyGram offices, not sure what to expect, but always cool under pressure. When the execs asked her to sing, she couldn't find a chair that would allow her to balance her guitar on her knee. They invited her to climb up on the conference room table, which she did, and by August 1994 Soraya had signed a major recording contract with Island/PolyGram Records and was scheduled for twin releases in English and Spanish.

HEIDI WEIDMAN
Soraya's United Airlines colleague and good friend

With candid excitement Soraya shared with me that the "right"
people had been given a demo tape. After that it all seemed like a
whirlwind. She quickly went from playing gigs at a small joint in
Coconut Grove and flying trips, to one day saying, "I got signed!!!"
I remember the call. You can't imagine the joy that I had, that we
all had. Our friend, our sweet talented friend, was now on her
path to fame. Early on in the process, Soraya and I agreed to let
our friendship remain void of fame. It sounds funny, but our
friendship had always just been based on giggles. Her singing, to
me, was always just icing on the cake of an incredible person.

MANOLO DIAZ
Then president of PolyGram Records

We called Soraya immediately, and days later we all sat in the conference room listening to her play her guitar and sing for more than two hours. We all fell in love as much with her as we had with her songs. This was why we decided to bet it all. Financed by PolyGram, we contracted with two prestigious British producers, Rod Argent and Peter Van Hook. Taking high risks with the talented young songwriter, we started a luxurious production at Abbey Road and elsewhere in London in 1995. Until then, all she had demonstrated was her professionalism as a flight attendant. Luckily for all of us, by 1997, Soraya's first album, recorded in both English and Spanish (a first in the industry), titled On Nights Like This/En Esta Noche, *had sold over a million copies worldwide. Suddenly a gigantic star was born.*

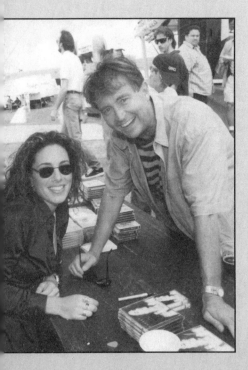

Once Soraya had a record deal, she needed a manager who could handle the business side so she could focus on being a musician. As a testament to Soraya's potential, she landed with the famous and flamboyant Miles Copeland, best known for being the longtime manager of the Police. Miles supported Soraya in her decision to focus on songwriting over performing, and he also put her in front of important audiences in Europe by pairing her with big-appeal artists like Sting and others for concerts, duets, and artistic collaboration.

◀ Soraya with Manolo Diaz on the road in 1996 promoting her first album.

PART TWO
THE RISE

Chapter 7

SOLO MI DIOS

I questioned my own strength and will of mind when I became a witness to my mother's illness. I would try to be strong when I went with her to the doctor, but I would always end up crying in my bathroom once we got back home. I was breaking inside, knowing I could do nothing to stop her pain.

She was the one to pull *me* through. In that way, she very much remained the mother, and I very much remained the child. By mere example, she would get me back on my feet again. A look, a touch of her hand was all I needed to know that there was a God and that love is exactly what I felt when I was with her.

Then true to her philosophy that life balances itself out, fate breathed her way and gave her a little room to rest. Surviving breast cancer for five years is considered a significant medical threshold. For some inexplicable yet beautiful reason, my mom reached her fifth year in remission while not undergoing any treatment. We were elated. She was overjoyed and reenergized. She told everyone, and, oh, how we celebrated.

But deep inside, the inexorable progression of the disease was marching to the beat of a drummer she could not see and could not control.

Just a few weeks later, she began to feel weak. She was vomiting again, although not from chemo, and overall, she was not looking well. Her skin tone was not right, her bones were hurting her terribly, and her breathing was getting short.

It all happened so fast. We went from celebrating to deciding whether to give her more treatment or just let her be. She went from being a cancer survivor to being terminally ill.

But the fighter she was, she would have none of that. The doctors were recommending that she give her body a rest, since the chemo would be too toxic for her and it had already proved ineffective. They had nothing else to offer her. But she refused.

"There must be something," she said, each time her voice getting stronger and stronger. What came from her next would mark me forever.

"Who are you to tell me that I am dying? *Solo mi Dios* . . . only my God knows when it is my time to come home, not you. You are a doctor, but you are only a man. Do *not* take away my hope."

"You are just a man," she would repeat to her doctor. "How can *you* tell me how much time I have?"

She was furious. She was also terrified.

In my frequent public speaking engagements, I repeat this to groups of survivors and at medical conventions. No one, no matter what the title, what the degree, can say for sure that you have x amount of time left in this world. And more important, no one has the right, no matter the intention, to take away a woman's sense of hope and her belief in the possibility that she might still recover.

The doctors relented, and she received more treatment. But as they had warned, it did nothing to thwart the cancer. There were no clinical trials for which she qualified, and all of the available chemotherapies had failed her. Still, she insisted.

"I don't want to just give up," she would plead. She charged ahead and held on to all she had left. Hope.

It was 1991 by then, but still, we did not have a lot of the treatments that we have now. She got sicker and sicker, until we finally asked her to stop. Her skin was already yellow from her failing liver, her pancreas was now affected by the cancer, and she was ever so weak.

On a little piece of yellow lined paper she wrote out her final wishes. She wrote that she was sorry she had to leave us. She asked us to place her in a specific hospice when she was ready. She then turned her attention to reconciling her fate and preparing to die.

Up until then, I had only a fear of death. The deep loss, the separation, the finality—I found all of it so frightening. The lessons she taught me continued beyond her demise.

It was 5:30 a.m. on Sunday, August 21, 1992. The cancer had the upper hand over my mom's body. For the last few days, she had been in a coma. We knew she was on her way to death, and all we could hope was that she would not suffer. We held on to any remaining chance that she might bounce back, until the doctors finally told us that they could do no more and that her vital signs and organs were beginning to fail her. That is when we decided to move her to hospice, not knowing how very brief her stay there would be. Her eyes were closed, and she was not responding to anything or to anyone. My dad and I were with her throughout the entire day, basically just sitting beside her bed, talking to her and making sure she was not in pain. My dad had been a wonderful caregiver for her, and now there was nothing more that he could do for her. She was being fed high doses of morphine intravenously, but she was breathing on her own. Her body was there, but we were unsure whether she had already left us.

That night my dad and I were getting ready to go home and get some rest, but as we were leaving something pulled me back. I asked my dad to wait a moment, and I went to talk to the head nurse.

"Can I sleep here tonight?"

"Sure you can, honey," she said with a slight southern drawl. "But your mom will be in good hands, you know. Why don't you just go home with your dad and get some rest," she insisted. "It's only her first night here and you should save your strength."

"Okay, but if I *want* to stay, can you help me set up a little cot?"

"Fine, dear. Give me a minute to get it set up for you."

I returned to my dad, who was waiting in the lobby.

"Dad, you go home. I've decided I'm going to spend the night. I don't know what, but something is not letting me leave."

"Are you sure?" he asked, red-eyed and tired.

"Yeah, no problem. They are going to set up a cot for me. I'll be fine. I'll call you if I need anything. I promise."

And with that he went home to rest, and I went back to my mom's room.

Finally, at about midnight, I rolled off into sleep. But before I did, I noticed a change in her breathing. All of a sudden, her breaths got louder and more intense. It almost sounded as if she had chest congestion. The cancer had spread to almost every organ in her body, including her lungs, so I just wrote off her heavy breathing to that. I got up to check on her. Her face seemed calm, so I kissed her good night on the forehead and got back into my little cot and closed my eyes.

At 5:20 a.m. I woke up abruptly, as if by a buzzing alarm clock. But the room was silent. I jumped out of the cot and slid on my socks over to my mom's bed. I sat down on the mattress with her.

Her breathing was even louder, and her chest moved awkwardly up and down. Then a few minutes later, as I held her hand in mine, it happened. It was just she and I in that room, and all you could hear was the clicking of the intravenous pump machine and her agitated breath.

She suddenly opened her eyes.

"Mámi, aquí estoy." *Mami, I am here.*

She looked right at me, and for those amazing seconds I saw the woman who had brought me into this world instead of the suffering body that had endured so much. Everything around me evaporated— her deteriorated body, the pump machines, my fond memories of the past, and my fearful thoughts of the future. It was just our eyes making contact.

I was speechless.

She turned her eyes upward, and as if she saw a familiar face, the corners of her mouth turned upward, and instantaneously the pained expression on her face morphed into a smile. Even the yellow tint of her skin flushed with a healthy pink hue.

I smiled back. For a split second I thought she was coming out of her coma and that at any moment, I would hear her voice continue to talk to me. This was the miracle I had been praying for.

Then a solitary tear rolled down from her right eye.

With that, she looked back down at me and closed her eyes again. The smile on her face remained. The clicking of the pump machine kept its time, but her breathing simply stopped.

What had she seen? Whom had she seen? I'll never know, of course. All I *do* know is that something happened that let her know it was her time and that it was all right for her to let go. I was left with the distinct impression that she left her suffering to go somewhere safe and familiar.

From that moment forward, I stopped fearing death. I knew she was whole again and I knew that she was not alone. I realized how much I believe that what dies is the body, but that the fire we all have rolling deep inside never goes out. Time is the gift, and everything else is on loan. All that is real is what we carry inside. I knew she had made peace and was resting.

As if I needed more assurance, she let me know later that night that all was well.

After a long morning calling relatives and talking with my dad at the hospice, I had returned home and taken a long, hot shower. As was my bad habit, I left my dirty clothes on the bathroom floor and melted into my bed, exhausted. The bathroom door was open and in clear view from my bed. Halfway through the night at around 3 a.m., I was awakened by my mom's voice. I thought I was dreaming. But she persisted until I actually woke up and sat up in my bed.

Without thinking about it, I answered back reflexively, "Ahh, I'll pick them up later, Mom. I was too tired when I got home."

"You have to get more organized now, okay?" she said, half joking.

There she was, standing in my bathroom picking up my clothes. She looked as she did before the cancer and the chemo took her apart piece by piece—beautiful, happy, and healthy.

Still half asleep, as I started to get up and walk toward her, it hit me. My mother is no longer of this earthly world. And she hasn't looked like this for the past few years.

"Sorayita, I am fine now," she said, holding the dirty clothes and coming toward me into the bedroom. "I don't want you to worry anymore. You have to be strong and take care of yourself. Remember you still have your *tias*. And take care of your father, please."

For the second time in twenty-four hours I was dumbfounded.

I nodded and then managed to get out a meager "O . . . o . . . okay, I promise."

So many things I wanted to ask her, so many things I wanted to tell her, but I could not string together a sentence. She smiled at me and disappeared into the air while moving down the hallway toward her room where my dad was sleeping. I wasn't spooked by this; in fact, I wasn't even perplexed, really—just amazed.

When I looked into my bathroom, I just started laughing aloud. The clothes she had been holding were no longer where I had left them on the bathroom floor. They were now on my bedroom floor, where she had stood talking to me.

On Nights Like This

No matter what anyone says time doesn't pull you through
Cause there are nights when I still cry when I think of you
Sometimes it swallows me in this space I feel inside
But I think of how strong you were and it helps me to get by

And all those nights when you would come to me in my dreams
I thought I was losing my mind, but it's the sanest I've ever been
And on those days, when life seems too much
I hear your voice and I'm comforted by your touch

On nights like this I know, that you're still here with me
On nights like this I know, you're in a better place
On nights like this I pray, I may be with you again someday
On nights like this I pray, that I may be
Worthy someday

There's the anger that blocked out the light
There's the doubts that held me captive night after night
The endless hours I spent asking why
When there's so many evil people, it just doesn't seem right

On nights like this I know, that you're still here with me
On nights like this I know, you're in a better place
On nights like this I pray, I may be with you again someday
On nights like this I pray, that I may be
Worthy someday

(continued)

On Nights Like This (continued)

And I remember the night when I held you in my arms
Trying to give you the strength, the will to hold on
And you looked in my eyes and said "Baby be strong,
I don't want to leave you but it's time for me to go"

And at that moment, as your hand slipped out of mine
A tear rolled down as you closed your eyes for the last time
And all the pain that had been written on your face
Suddenly disappeared and by a smile it was replaced

On nights like this I know, that you're still here with me
On nights like this I know, you're in a better place
On nights like this I pray, I may be with you again someday
On nights like this I pray, that I may be
Worthy someday

Chapter 8

MUSIC LESSONS

We are all born with unique abilities and talents. These gifts somehow reveal themselves when we need them most. Sometimes we apply these talents subconsciously; sometimes, as in my case, you are born with an innate awareness that you've been given something that's bigger than yourself. For me it was music. As a child I took only a handful of guitar lessons. After a few, I told my dad to save his money because I could figure it out on my own. I would watch guitarists on television and copy how they moved their hands. I would sit for hours listening over and over again to the recordings of my favorite artists, and I would study how they would rhyme their lyrics, what chords they would use and how their melodies would weave in and out of their stories. I would listen to each until I had broken the code.

This was my first step toward becoming a songwriter. I spent hours doing this as a child. Nothing made me feel happier than that moment when it snapped into place in my head and I "saw" the music come to life. Nothing before or since has ever made me feel so connected. It was a language all my own, and at an early age I reveled in being able to fully immerse myself in it.

Instead of daydreaming about princes and faraway adventures, I daydreamed about musical notes. The notes just appear in my head, literally. Sometimes I see them alone, sometimes in layers, and always in constant movement. It is as if I have my own language, a private lexicon that draws me further and further into myself. As a child, I did not feel the need to develop outwardly when my music would take me higher than any playdate with a friend or any story in a book. First the music flowed forth from my brain like a slightly muddy river. I'd often dam it up by playing and singing what I heard. I'd write it down. Then I would embellish a word here and there, change a chord, and modify the melody until the water from the new stream was clear and pure. As I began to bring the music down from my head into my hands and let it flow out onto the guitar strings and through the air in my lungs, I realized I had stumbled upon my own little piece of heaven. I had found my purpose. Since then, other than at the times when my illness wouldn't let me, no more than one day has gone by without me sitting down with my guitar and at least just holding it. The feeling of the wood in the palm of my left hand, the exquisite curve that sits perfectly under my right arm, the vibration of the strings that my fingers can manipulate with my eyes closed—this entire sensory experience awakens something deep within my soul.

People have often asked how I write songs, and it's not an easy thing to describe. I see the notes before I even hear them. One by one they come, followed by the harmonies. When I was younger, I did not know what any of it was called, I just knew what it looked like. It floated around in my head like kites on a windy day. Then I would sit down, close my eyes, and turn the wispy choruses and verses in my head into complete songs of my own. Then, and still now, the songs and words have colors and I see them blending together. They fall into place like a colored matrix.

This is the moment of creation for me, and it is like nothing else I have ever felt. Word by word, it just starts to flow, and it's a struggle for my scribbling to keep up with my visions. As I play the chords on the guitar and start to hum the melody with my voice, I hear the string arrangement, or the bass line, or the notes the backup vocalists are singing. It is almost too much stimuli, but I don't try to block it or slow it down. I am open, I am a conduit, and I try to stay in this zone for as long as I can or until the torrent in my mind stops on its own. It feels like this every single time. Writing music is not a job for me, but rather a privilege of which I am very aware.

Music is not entertainment for me. It is pure bliss. It is a direct line to my faith. Creating something so beautiful from nothing has taught me that I am much more than just flesh and bones. Being a musician planted tools within me that would be needed later on in my life. Music, contrary to what most of us think when we think of pop stars, has actually taken me *away* from my ego. It has shown me that the more honest I am with my true self, the more I open up my heart and mind, the more prolific and creative I will be. When I humbly let those musical vibrations flow and find their own path in and around what-ever might be happening and bouncing around in me at that particular moment, that is when I get that precious feeling.

Even when listening to live or recorded music, I tend to break it apart. If it is "good," I feel it. I feel the air in the singer's voice or the movement of the bow on the violin strings. I envision where the com-poser was when he or she wrote the piece. I am transported to a true state of extrasensory perception. A slightly out-of-tune string sounds like nails on a chalkboard to me, and sometimes an easy, poorly writ-ten verse unravels the entire song in just a few syllables and I am no longer able to enjoy it.

Silence, on the other hand, has a melody all its own. For me, silence is a true connection to my spirit. The notes I will sing or play come from this silence and are therefore an extension of my soul. It is this silence that links it all together and gives me the hints as to what the emotion is behind that melody. That is how I can understand a com-poser and his or her intention. When I sing, I feel not just the lyric, I sing not just the melody, but I become both. I bring into every word and every note all that I am. Today I might sing a certain way, but if I were to sound exactly the same tomorrow, I would not be true to my art. A song is alive and forever changing because the person who is interpreting it is alive and brings that vibrancy into the performance.

Having had this with me all of my life made meditation and mind control an easy, and almost logical, next step for me. This inner world became my world, and I became totally accustomed to solitary pursuits. I was used to silence, and I was comfortable with being alone with myself and with my thoughts. For much of what I would have to deal with in fighting cancer, I had been practicing all of my life.

Music has taught me much more than just how to play a song and how to sing. Music taught me patience. Sometimes you have to wait for the right melody or the right word before you can complete your song. Music taught me teamwork. When you are playing as a part of a band or an orchestra or a quartet, you have to be aware of your place among the others and know when to stand out and when to support. Music taught me the value of dedication. The more you play and the more you repeat a work, the better you get. Not just in terms of skill, but with enough repetition, you start to listen differently and you begin to hear the music that falls into the silences between the notes you are playing. Little did I know how much I would use patience, teamwork, and dedication in my fight against cancer.

Although I am often asked to write a song for a particular artist or soundtrack, I approach this part of my life without pressure and without specific goals. If I cannot come up with a word, a story, a melody, or even a chord, I let it go and walk away. I know and trust that it will come. Sure enough, it is usually at the most random and inconvenient moments that the light goes on and I take that first step toward creation. Soon enough it is done.

This part of my career has also taught me to accept assignments that truly inspire me. Because without inspiration there can be no imagination. And without imagination, the soul gets stuck. Many a time I have found my wings through song. My mantras during meditation are sometimes melodic, sometimes just the rhythm of my breath. Either way, if I am troubled or encumbered by the events of the day or the weight of life's never-ending challenges, I call out to those angels and hop on their wings. Even in the middle of a loud, noisy, crowded room, I can rise above the clamor and find my own altitude filled with peace and warm vibrancy.

So much of this has allowed me to simply have a place to go when everything around me seems to be shattering and falling down on top of me. I can retreat into this world that offers me both protection and an outlet for working out the deepest of emotional challenges.

Music always served as a bond between my parents and me. When I was about ten years old, my father worked out an arrangement with Mr. Carroll. He was an older retired man who taught violin. My dad would come home from work after a long commute, grab a quick bite to eat, then drive me to my lessons. He would sit just outside the open door and listen to our playing. I had excelled beyond the school's music program, so my dad found Mr. Carroll through a friend's recommendation. Sometimes we could not pay the full cast of the lesson, but once Mr. Carroll heard me play and saw how dedicated I was, he would sometimes give me a lesson for free.

He would give me extremely difficult assignments, and yet I would practice until the skin under my jaw was raw and my fingertips were sore. He would tease me by saying that if I were only a better player and if I were older he would let me play in his quartet. Ever since the night that my dad and I stopped by during one of their performances, I was captivated: four retired professional classical musicians playing the masterpieces. Heaven. Even though I was only ten, I asked him what I had to do to earn his invitation. He gave me the stock answer: Practice, practice, practice!

I did, and it paid off when he finally invited me to play second violin with his quartet, sitting in for one of the regulars who had something else to do that night. He knew that their musical selection of Vivaldi's *Four Seasons* was not only part of my own repertoire but was one of my favorites. I had memorized both the first and second violin parts and was truly ready to go. I arrived incredibly nervous. My mom came along to Mr. Carroll's that night for the first time, and because of this special moment, my parents sat inside the rehearsal room instead of out in the hall. Always ready with a braid for any occasion, she had done my hair in an intricate French version and had bought me new shoes. My mom wore a dress with some beautiful jewelry—Lebanese gold and Colombian emeralds that once belonged to her mother. My father usually took off his coat and tie when he got home from work and rushed to get me to violin class. On this night, he stayed fully dressed in his best clothes.

I was screaming with excitement inside, but I held myself together in front of these musicians. I knew the score like the back of my hand, so even at age ten I was telling myself I just had to stay calm, be patient, and fall into the music. It was spectacular. At first the men looked at me with skepticism; I could sense their compassion but I knew that there would be a limit to their tolerance. After we played the first "Season," everything changed. I had been playing the entire piece with my eyes closed. My passion was guiding me and I was locked into that inner world that I held so dear. When we were through, and I finally opened my eyes, they were staring at me with an incredulous look on their faces. If I could allow myself an immodest moment, it was a flawless performance. Mr. Carroll just smiled and the others shook my hand as if I were a grown-up. My parents were beaming. They had heard me practice that piece hour after hour in our little apartment. My father had even gotten me a recording of a quartet with which I played time and time again like an early form of violin karaoke.

After that night Mr. Carroll suggested that my parents allow me to audition for the Youth Symphony Orchestra of New York. He felt it would prepare me for what he saw as my next step: an audition to join the famed Juilliard School of Music. I practiced for another year or so and by the time I was twelve, I was playing the Mendelssohn Violin Concerto. Mr. Carroll knew I was ready.

We took the train into Manhattan one rainy Sunday afternoon. As I walked into the audition room, I realized I was the youngest one there. All the other musicians seemed like pros, and for a split second I thought I was in the wrong place. My mom squeezed my hand and reminded me in her broken English that I was ready and if they decided not to accept me it would be their loss.

I took out my violin, tuned it, rosined my bow, went over my musical selection once more in my head, and waited for my name to be called. A couple of weeks later, I was officially named a member of the New York City Youth Symphony Orchestra.

We played many concerts, but none would ever outshine my first at Carnegie Hall. I was twelve, and I asked my parents to take me there quite early. Luckily, as we were tiptoeing around trying to find ways for me to get comfortable, we ran into a Hispanic member of the hall staff whom they convinced to let us in and up onto that stage. I will never forget that moment. My mom and dad were the only two souls in the audience, and I heard every crack of the old wood as I walked to center stage. It was such a big place and I was so small, and yet I was completely and utterly at home. Once the concert started, the earlier visit spared me the nerves I would have had. I looked around, took a deep breath, lifted my instrument to my chin, and played like I had never played before. The suspicion I had about myself as a performer was confirmed: I was a person who could gain such complete control over my nerves that I could focus on the audience and what *they* needed. I knew I had found my place. Now I just had to keep working to earn it.

The Carnegie Hall experience resonated within me for years. Instead of being afraid of the big stage, I felt drawn to it, and some of my happiest moments stem from that day: being on stage with Sting, sitting around my living room jamming with amazing musicians, opening my eyes after singing a song and seeing the expressions on the people's faces in the audience.

Music was a part of my essence from an early age, but as a grown woman, it has provided a shield for me. As a grown woman, that solitary little girl is still a part of me. When I am with my guitar, whether I am home or onstage in front of thousands, I am suspended in my own universe. At times throughout my life, and particularly before my diagnosis, people perceived me as aloof, but in reality I have always found comfort in that piece of myself that needs to process things on her own time and in her own way, regardless of public opinion.

Since my diagnosis, I have changed, but my fundamental nature is still the same. I hold on to that borderline stubbornness that does not allow me to give up, even when the odds are stacked against me. I do have more of a need now to connect on different levels with different kinds of people—I often feel that I have something I need to say. So I seek out public forums in which I can communicate and make those connections, and I am often out and about meeting people, speaking publicly, doing both the business of music and the business of being a patient advocate. All the while, of course, I must go about being a patient myself. But this is new. The part of me that I truly understand is the one that likes to think, likes to be alone, loves intellectual and artistic challenges, and is convinced that it is not how far you get but how you live along the way that matters. It is the pursuit of living the way that is best for me, and the comfort that comes from having the confidence to know what that is, that has guided me throughout the battles with my own body.

Chapter 9

HEIGHTS AND DEPTHS

By the year 2000, I had already recorded and released two CDs, each of them in both English and Spanish, and I was on the verge of my third worldwide release. All the risks I had taken—flying for United instead of pursuing a career more in keeping with my education, singing in coffeehouses and basically anyplace that would give me a microphone—had paid off. I had a major recording contract with Universal/PolyGram and number-one charting songs, and I had tasted touring success with live concerts throughout the United States, Latin America, and Europe. Between my debut in 1996 and 2000, my life had changed radically. I had played in front of seventy-five thousand people and gotten stuck crossing borders in Europe. I had learned the difference between fans who truly "get" my music and the kind who would tie themselves to my tour bus to ask for my hand in marriage. There were hair people and makeup people and people custom-sewing stage clothes for me. I was desperately trying to find spare time in every day to keep running so I would look good in those clothes!

It was an exciting time in the music industry, and I got to experience those glamorous days. I was managed by Miles Copeland, the famed manager of the Police and Sting, with whom I got to tour. I also played and toured with Michael Bolton, Natalie Merchant, Alanis Morissette, and other greats. I was fortunate that the record company had genuine faith in me, because they were pushing me hard. They gave me the privilege of working with producing legends from the British world like Rod Argent and Peter Van Hook and having my music videos produced by people like Matt Mahurin, the well-known director of videos for U-2, Metallica, Peter Gabriel, and Sting. As a result, in much of Latin America and in a number of European countries, I had become a household name, and the press featured me pretty consistently. It was crazy but it was fun, and it was bigger than my parents would ever have dared to dream.

One of the hardest things for me was not being able to share all this with my mom. Her absence lingers in my head and pulses heavy in my heart every time something glorious occurs in my life. I know she would have loved my work. She never heard my music on the radio, never saw me on talk shows, never watched her *telenovelas* only to hear my music accompanying them. I think of the night I walked the red carpet in Los Angeles and won a Grammy, and with an empty ache I think about what it would have been like to have had her there with me. She always dreamed of traveling to faraway places like Hawaii, and now that I can finally afford to take her there, she's not here. How she would have loved to sit in my garden. More than anything, how she would have loved to see that she *did* do a very good job raising me.

My music served as the passport to a world our family could barely imagine, and I know my mom would have been the perfect partner for this adventure. I missed her deeply. But by 2000, my life was on a good path, and I was finally finding my light after her death. Inside, I had grown, and I was becoming the woman I had always wanted to be.

Then life decided that it was time to shift gears. In May of 2000, everything as I knew it began to change. Here I began to understand that I was not the master of my own destiny.

I had flown to Cali, Colombia, to visit my *tia* America. Like my mom years before, and like her mother, she was dying of breast cancer. We all have a favorite relative, and she was mine. When we lived in Colombia, I was literally her shadow.

America was elegant and stunning, with her lavender Elizabeth Taylor eyes. She was undoubtedly the matriarch of this generation of my family, a role she adopted without hesitation after her own mother, my *abuela* Nayibe, died. I was fascinated by the way she managed her own business, ran her household, and basically took care of everyone. She was the living embodiment of a proud, self-confident woman, and I breathed in every ounce of her determination and independence.

Nothing was impossible for her, and I know this is where my ambitious spirit came from. She started working at a very young age, but the path to her eventual financial success was filled with obstacles both large and small. It is worth noting that hers was not an easy personality. She was quite demanding not only of herself but of her family as well. Her marriage was difficult, and although it was easy to be her niece, I suspect it must have been harder to be her child. She took care of things for her children instead of letting them do it themselves, and at the same time she expected them to be independent. Everything revolved around her and depended upon her. Yet even during the toughest times, I would flip through pictures of her and see her posing elegantly in beautiful dresses, matching shoes, and perfectly coiffed hair. She always seemed so together and so unafraid.

She was also just like her mother and grandmother, generous and charitable. In addition to the countless gifts she gave to family and strangers alike, her generous spirit is exemplified by what she eventually decided to do with her dream home. She and her family had built this hacienda from the ground up. At one point, I was even there to help lay the tile floor in the porch. She tended to every plant and loved to walk the enormous grounds and inspect the citrus and avocado trees. She created an oasis where the entire extended family and friends would always gather. The dream home I eventually designed in Miami is a Colombian hacienda inspired by the one she had built years before just outside of Cali.

But her forty-six-year-old husband, Guillermo, died suddenly during a birthday party in his honor at their home, and the hacienda became a painful reminder of one of the worst events in her life. Although it was worth a tremendous amount of money, she pretty much gave it away to a group of nuns from the United States who would later turn it into a school for young children. Her behavior perplexed many, but it did not surprise me in the least. These nuns became her friends and she would confide in them things she would never discuss with any of us. Serendipitously, one of my *tia*'s granddaughters would eventually be a student at the school that was once her home.

In light of all of this and more, my *tia* was perfect in my eyes.

I decided to make the trip to Colombia in May 2000, when I received a phone call from my uncle. My *tia*'s cancer had completely invaded her body, all of the treatments had stopped working, and now they were just draining her lungs to help her keep breathing and trying to ease the excruciating pain in her bones with radiation. She had told my uncle that she was ready to let go, and that's when I got the phone call.

I had been her confidante throughout her diagnosis, either in person, over the phone, or through letters. She had known for years that something was wrong. A part of me believes that when she flew down to south Florida to help us with my mom's new townhome years earlier, she already knew she was ill. But for many complicated reasons, she never got a mammogram or went to the doctor. In a strange way, while everyone else was mad at her for her lack of action, I understood her. She had seen her mother mutilated by surgeons. She had held her mother's hand while she threw up. She had knitted caps for her bald head. She had held her while she cried from the discomfort of the treatments. She had helped her clean the scar across her chest. Ultimately, she saw her succumb to a quick and painful death. Who in her right mind would rush off to the doctor to learn for certain that the same fate was about to befall her? Perhaps for my aunt, a few years of ignorant bliss was the ticket to the highest-quality existence, for *her*. I can't condone it, particularly since treatments can now be truly life-enhancing and life-extending. But I can understand it.

I am convinced my aunt believed that treatments would not really help her buy any more time. I think she had complete faith that she would eventually die, and if that was going to be the outcome either way, then it might as well be on her terms, so she let it be. Until she could not handle the pain.

When she finally chose to go see her doctor, the unchecked cancer had already broken through her skin. The tumors were like balls across her chest, and the cancer had already metastasized to her lungs, bones, and liver.

In vain, at this point, but at the insistence of her doctor, she decided she would undergo treatment. Basically, the pain was so severe that she gave in to the young oncologist who was trying everything he could to buy her more time. Nothing worked, of course. The cancer continued to grow and spread. They enrolled her in a clinical trial, and that seemed to stabilize her for a few months, but that eventually stopped working as well.

I remember being with her during this last trip and preparing her medications. She was explaining to me that one pill was for the bone pain, but that the other one was a clinical trial drug. It was some new type of chemotherapy that she could take in pill form and would not cause her hair to fall out. She proudly mentioned that the drug was not yet available in the United States and that they had chosen a few women for a test to see whether it worked. She knew she did not have much time left, and she chose to do this for the same reason she did so many other things in her life—she had nothing to lose and maybe she would be helping other women in the future. Little did she know back then that the one she would be helping would be me.

The dosage was still not right, so her side effects were unpredictable. One that stood out in my mind was that the soles of her feet and the palms of her hands swelled and turned a deep purple. Years later, in my own battle with breast cancer, my doctor prescribed me a drug newly approved by the FDA. Possible side effects included "hand and foot syndrome," which sounded exactly like what my aunt experienced with that swelling and discoloration. When I saw the pill, I recognized it as the same one that I prepared for my *tia* years earlier. My aunt was an early test subject, and I, along with tens, or even hundreds, of thousands of women years later would benefit from her willingness. Breast cancer has been like a tornado that's cut a deadly swath through our family, but somehow a few positive things have been delivered by its winds. This drug is one of them. It kept my cancer in remission for over a year with minimal side effects. My quality of life was spectacular, and every time I took that little pill I thought of my aunt and gave her a quiet prayer of appreciation.

But the purpose of my rushed visit at the end of May of 2000 was to say good-bye to this glorious woman. I spent the entire flight crying quietly in my seat. After being by my mom's side and watching the cancer take her away eight years earlier, I was not sure how I was going to be able to handle seeing my *tia* facing the same extraordinary circumstances. The ride from the airport to her home seemed to take forever. Once I arrived, I had to pause and take a deep breath before I could enter her apartment.

I opened the door to find her sitting in her favorite chair. She was a ghost of the woman she once was. She had on her pajamas, and only a few strands of hair were on her beautiful head. When she saw me, a magnificent smile spread over her face. My instinct was to run up to her and give her a huge, long, warm hug, but I knew from experience that her frail body could not handle such contact. Breast cancer and its treatments often have the effect of making one's skin so sensitive that the patient can't bear the sensation of even a warm breeze. I stopped short and tenderly kissed her on the forehead, knelt down by her side, and just held her hands in mine.

She told me she had been waiting up for me and asked if I would help her get to bed. We shuffled to her bedroom. My heart and mind were spinning. When I helped her lie down, I got a glimpse of her chest and what I saw made my world crumble. She was covered in tumors. Her chest wall had huge lumps everywhere. Breast cancer most frequently metastasizes to the bones, liver, brain, and lungs, and as a result her breathing was forced and her skin had taken on a yellow hue, thin and translucent. Her body was shutting down. She knew it. We all knew it. She asked me to pray with her, then she asked me to promise to take care of myself and to keep an eye on another aunt of mine,

Stella. Stella had not only come to Boca Raton to help take care of my mom, but she had also been America's primary caregiver.

Then she told me how proud she was of me. In a way, I heard my mom through her. My mom was not able to see my success as a musician, but *tia* America did. She, not my mom, was able to see me grow into womanhood. It was very special to receive that kind of validation from the woman I had always wanted to emulate. I told her she was my hero and how proud I was to be her niece. Then her eyes slowly began to close and she wandered off into sleep. I stayed with her for a while, then I had to step away. The emotion was too strong and I could not handle any more. I went into the room where I was staying and regained my composure. Then I joined the rest of the family in the living room.

I was to spend barely three days with her. I had just released my third CD, *Cuerpo y Alma*, with its English counterpart, *I'm Yours*, on the way. In the music business this is a hectic time of interviews and promotions, and I needed to get back to work. The record company had generously given me time off to take this important trip, but I had to get back, and three days was all I had.

On the second day of my visit, as I was taking a shower, I noticed a bump under my left arm. As the day progressed, I felt my left breast start to itch and feel strange. At the end of the day, as I was changing into my pajamas, I was shocked to see that my breast was turning very red and swollen. Whatever this was, it was getting worse by the hour. It was a Friday.

I did not know what to do. I stood there in the bathroom, staring into the mirror, and I began to sweat and feel dizzy. I could not tell anyone there. There was just too much fear and loss pervading the family, and we all had to stay focused on making my aunt comfortable. But what in the world was happening? This is just ridiculous. *God, what are you doing?!*

I called my closest friend in Miami and told her what I had just found. Without skipping a beat, she begged me not to worry and said that she would call my doctor and get an appointment for the following Monday.

Leaving my *tia* was incredibly difficult. Saying a permanent good-bye to another beautiful woman was more than I could bear. I cursed the cancer; I cursed life for being so unfair. I urged the family to try to reduce her suffering as much as possible. But even giving her morphine proved to be difficult, since her veins were almost completely collapsed. She could no longer lie down, sit up, or walk, as the pain in her bones was so severe. She told me that even the air hurt as it touched her skin. I kissed her good-bye and for the first time told her what my mom had said just as she died. I told her to look for her and to have faith that soon her pain would go away forever. I asked again if there was anything I could do for her, but she barely shook her head and whispered that she was not afraid.

I got back home on Saturday, and it was without a doubt the longest weekend of my life. My heart was so heavy from what I had just experienced with my *tia*, and yet I had this weird thing happening in my body that I could not and did not want to understand. Just six months earlier I had had a full checkup, including a mammogram, and I was fine. I shared what was happening to my body with another good friend, and we convinced ourselves that maybe it was an infection of some sort, or that maybe some strange bug had bitten me during my trip. Everything was an option except the big white elephant in the room. That would just be too much. Life could not be so cruel.

Chapter 10

HOW DO I?

As soon as I returned from Colombia after saying good-bye to my *tia* America, I had to deal with this mysterious lump under my arm. Monday came around, and I nervously made my way to the doctor's office. He asked to see what was going on, felt around under my arm, and in less than five minutes asked me to go ahead and get dressed. He would be right back, he said. "Right back" turned into twenty minutes. He came back into the consultation room and told me that he had taken the liberty of calling a doctor friend of his who had agreed to see me right away.

I barely had time to take this in, but I somehow got out the words "What does that mean, Doc?"

He looked so solemn, it was surreal when he spoke: "What is happening with your breast and under your arm just does not feel right to me and I do not want to waste any time. I need you to go see a specialist."

He wrote down an address and told me to go right over; they were waiting for me. *Waiting, for me?*

I arrived, stood outside the door, and processed the words on the door. "Oncological surgeon." My knees gave.

Even though the office was filled with patients, as soon as I checked in, one of the nurses immediately came out to get me. I was moved into a room with a long table and asked to remove my top and bra and put on an uncomfortably rough peach-colored paper gown. Why the mind remembers unimportant details like that I do not understand. In just a few minutes, I was meeting the man who was to become my new doctor. He introduced himself, although I did not hear a word or even catch his name. He began asking me some questions, and as I tried to answer, my voice kept cracking. Then he began the examination, and after what seemed like only seconds, he asked me to sit up and he pulled over a chair.

He began to explain to me what a biopsy is. He explained what a needle aspiration is. *Of course I know these terms, I sat with my mom during this same conversation with her surgeon,* I thought to myself, not fully grasping that he was talking about me, about my body. Then he began to explain to me that it was very important that he perform a biopsy right now in this room. He would numb the area and then stick a small needle into the masses he was feeling under my arm and in my breast. I would not feel any pain, he promised.

I was at a loss. I began to cry, more out of confusion than anything else. He put his arms around me and just told me to be strong right now, and at that point I realized what a wonderful doctor I had ended up with. We had to do this to find out what was going on inside of my body, he said. My family history of breast cancer was too strong not to take this seriously, he said. He asked that I trust him when he said that it would not hurt. But at no point did he say, "I don't think it's anything serious." That was the only thing I wanted to hear him say.

He was right, the biopsy didn't hurt. Not getting the answer right away did. I was stupefied. My knees were shaking as I walked back to the car. When I got home, I could not make the key open the door, and I broke down in frustration and terror at the threshold of my sanctum.

I tried to eat, but I had no appetite. My best friends gathered around me. Miami was so far from my real family that a few close friends had become my lifeline throughout the years. We have been a part of each other's lives for years and they have been by my side through all sorts of rough seas; we now consider each other family. Together they tried to take away some of my burden, but my mind was just too hazy.

"He'll call tomorrow. There's nothing else you can do today," they kept saying.

A few hours later, the phone rang.

"Are you alone?" the doctor asked.

"No, my buddies are here."

"Good. Soraya, I received the results of the pathology of the needle biopsy we did today. I wanted to talk to you in person, but I want to make sure that we get moving first thing in the morning, so I need you to know this now. Are you all right with speaking to me over the phone?"

"Yeah, sure, I guess," I stumbled.

"It looks like the mass in your breast is cancer. Furthermore, before we can go any further and before an oncologist can start working with me on a treatment plan, we need to get a better tumor sample and check out the tumor under your arm. I want you to . . . *blah* . . . *blah* . . . *blah* . . . are you understanding me?"

"Actually, no. I am so confused right now."

"Okay, just grab a pen and paper and write this down," he said.

I began scribbling . . . tomorrow . . . hospital . . . morning . . . no food . . . biopsy . . . anesthesia . . . outpatient . . . later schedule bone scan . . . PET scan . . . CAT scan . . . check organs . . . size of tumor . . . stage of disease . . . chemo . . . surgery . . . radiation . . .

He went on and on, but the only thing that echoed in my head was CANCER.

I hung up the phone.

I have breast cancer.

How could that be?

I ran three miles a day, I ate well, I lived a good, clean life with no bad habits, no addictions. I had made some mistakes, I took wrong turns sometimes, I made some bad decisions, but overall, I was a pretty decent human being. Why did this feel like a punishment? How could life be so cruel? Our family had suffered so much already at the hands of this disease.

My surgeon's voice haunted me. I have breast cancer.

I was thirty-one years old.

I could not get up the nerve to call my father. How would I tell him?

"Call him, Sori. We are right here for you," my friends urged.

They dialed the phone for me because I suddenly could not remember his phone number. I heard his voice and began to cry. I gathered my breathing and began again.

"Papi, I . . . I . . . went to the doctor today and um . . . well . . ."

I couldn't say it.

"Come on, Sori, you need to say this aloud. He needs to know," said my friends.

"Papi, I have to go to the hospital tomorrow morning."

Silence on the other end.

"Um . . . I . . . They . . . they say that I have breast cancer, Dad. . . . I . . . need to have a biopsy right away."

Silence.

"Dad?"

Silence.

"Dad!!?"

"But they say you are going to be fine, no?" he asked in a broken voice.

"No, Dad, I haven't heard that yet. It seems pretty serious."

"But are they sure? You are so young, Sorayita, are they sure?"

"Well, that's what we are going to find out tomorrow."

"You are going to be fine. You will be fine."

I heard his tears over the phone.

"Dad, I have to go. No, don't come now, it's late. See me tomorrow after I get back home."

That was the hardest phone call of my life. Like my mom, I worried more about him than me at that point.

The next morning I went to the hospital, and as I was recovering from the biopsy, the surgeon went to speak to my "family." He was brutally honest with them. Years later I would find out they had asked him to spare me the full extent of his prognosis, fearing it would drain all of the hope out of me. I'm thankful for that. He told them that the cancer was aggressive and that it would be hard to fully eliminate. He told them the treatment would be difficult beyond comprehension and that my chances for survival beyond the treatment were dismal. And that even if I made it past the initial treatments, at some point in the future I would most probably be dealing with a recurrence even stronger than this time around.

After I recovered from the anesthesia, the prognosis he gave me was gentler, but still, it painted a bleak picture of what lay ahead for me. He told me that I had to be a fighter. That I had to give it all I had because this damn thing was going to be hard to beat. That he promised to do everything to help me, but I had to be more courageous than I ever thought I could be. Still, I can only imagine what he would have said if he had not been asked to censor his words.

And so, on June 6, 2000, my new life began.

Two weeks later I received a phone call from Colombia. My *tia* had died in her sleep. She was sixty-four.

I decided from that moment forward that I would stop asking, "Why me?" and start asking, "How do I?"

I approached every chemotherapy treatment as if it would get me one step closer to healthy. Since I was strong and young, they gave me drugs that were tough. But it had to be that way. The damned cancer was a formidable challenge, and I was determined not to let it get the best of me. It was during this time that I evolved beyond what I thought was my capability. Once I accepted my reality, all of that energy was freed up to be channeled in another direction.

One of the advantages of being the fourth person in your family to face this diagnosis is that the lack of predetermined treatment protocols was not a surprise to me. Unlike heart disease, diabetes, or so many other things, even certain types of cancer, there just isn't any one way to treat breast cancer. The doctors have to "try" things. I decided to place inordinate faith in them. But we would be a team. Having been through it with my mother, I understood that I had to be active in my treatment and help choose the combination of therapies that would most likely have the best effect. I had to do research. I had to ask questions. I had to find specialists in whom I could place my trust. And each of those decisions felt as if it was of life-or-death magnitude. I *had* to channel all my energy toward healing; there was no choice about it.

That meant putting down my music. In my career, I was just about to start traveling Latin America and Europe, promoting my new CD and performing. But visits to radio stations, other interviews, and performances were immediately canceled. For the first time in my life, I even stopped writing songs. I was focused one hundred percent on my healing.

I have breast cancer. I cannot change that. It is not my fault. My life will never go back to what it was. I, not the cancer, will define myself. I repeated these things to myself over and over; it became a powerful mantra. Without it, I would have never found solid ground. Slowly and painfully, I worked my way through the sequence of treatments.

Reflection

Beauty's only skin deep, they say it fades away with time
I promise I will search for you, and find you deep inside
Flowers are so radiant when they are in bloom
But seasons betray them, stealing their perfume

I hear you when the wind blows
I see you in a summer sun
I feel you with my beating heart
You are my reflection
In your eyes I am beautiful
Imperfections were never such a charm

Stones are often hidden, buried out of sight
On them we can build up straight to the sky
When we are together it's unabashed and tender
Funny how love feels when it's made of sweet surrender

I hear you when the wind blows
I see you in a summer sun
I feel you with my beating heart
You are my reflection
In your eyes I am beautiful
Imperfections were never such a charm

Falling into silence it unravels in my mind
Thoughts appear like flowing clouds moving without time
Rivers will flow straight into the sea
If you believe in that then you believe in me

(continued)

Reflection (continued)

I hear you when the wind blows
I see you in a summer sun
I feel you with my beating heart
You are my reflection
In your eyes I am beautiful
Imperfections were never such a charm

Chapter 11

AN ARMY FOR CHANGE

fter my initial diagnosis in June 2000, after the dust settled, after all of the tests and scans, after all the second and third opinions and all of the other craziness, some clear, frightening thoughts broke through to my consciousness: I was going to lose my hair, lose my energy, lose my breasts. And although I kept swatting it away like a pesky fly, there was the fear that I might lose my life.

On the career side, the promotion machine was in full swing for my new CD, and I was scheduled to leave home for many months.

But now I had cancer.

One calm afternoon, in the middle of tests and scans, I did what I had not done in years. I plopped myself down on the couch and turned on the television and did some channel surfing. For years I had been traveling so much and working so hard that the last thing I wanted to do during my free time was to watch television. But this particular afternoon I was trying to distract myself because my head was just too tired from all of the thought traffic it had been trying to control.

I stopped on one of the Spanish-language channels. Not even two weeks had passed since my biopsy. I was getting scan and test results back, and we were finalizing plans for my treatment with everyone involved. I had not yet told my record company what was going on, as I was a long way from going public with this information. I simply told them I needed a little more time off after the visit to Colombia to say good-bye to *tia*.

My health was private. It was my life and no one else's business. But as I was flipping channels that day, I caught a glimpse of my picture on one of those gossipy talk shows. I thought they were going to mention my new CD and show the new video that we had just recorded in Canada, but no. Someone who did not know me, whom I had never met, decided to take it upon himself to say that I had been diagnosed with breast cancer, that I was in extremely poor health, and that the prognosis was not good.

At first I was in shock. Then I got angry.

Actually, it was much worse than anger. I was fuming: How dare they treat this like a rumor about a romance or a speeding ticket or a temper outburst caught on tape!?! This was *my life*.

I picked up the phone and called my team over. We had to have a plan. I needed to focus *completely* on healing my body, and I did not have the time or the energy to deal with this stuff. I needed their support and their guidance.

I also decided to call my friends at the Susan G. Komen Foundation. In fact, it was Nancy Brinker, the sister of Susan Komen and the founder of the foundation, who would be my lifeline during these crucial first steps in confronting my diagnosis and prognosis.

Nancy and I had met earlier that year at a fund-raiser on a Spanish television network. I had always been very vocal about early detection and mammograms and had shared my mom's struggle during interviews. I always thought that if I could use my fame to spotlight this subject, which was somewhat awkward or even taboo for Latinas at that time, I would be doing some good. The record companies didn't always like it, but I felt it was important to speak substance in an industry that is built on shallow fluff.

In preparation for that fund-raiser, the TV network had asked if I would perform the song that I wrote for my mom, and the paperwork came over to my team. Usually the producers of the show ask for a rider, which is like a contract full of the performer's special requests. Many performers will request a limo, a private dressing room, a certain type of catering, and even crazy things to satisfy crazy cravings. I asked, instead, to have five minutes with Nancy Brinker. Nothing more, nothing less. I had discovered the Susan G. Komen Breast Cancer Foundation through their Race for the Cure events, and it was at these gatherings that I had found comfort in realizing that I was not alone. Wearing my mom's name pinned to the back of my race T-shirts, I met other motherless daughters, and, more important, I met survivors. I could not believe how many there were! I felt that I had found a place where I could take all of the loss I felt inside and turn it around. It was the Susan G. Komen Breast Cancer Foundation and their outreach events that helped me realize I could be more than a casualty. I could be a part of the solution!

At this fund-raiser in early 2000, I had wanted to personally thank Nancy for that, and also to offer her my voice as a link to the Spanish media. As in other minority communities, it was becoming clear that Latina women did not practice breast self-exams or have regular clinical checkups, nor did they understand the importance of yearly mammograms to the degree that they should. I was going to be on the road in the upcoming months promoting my new CD, and what a great opportunity to include this in my speaking points during interviews.

We met briefly that night and followed it up with a beautiful lunch during which a friendship and mutual understanding blossomed. Nancy had not only suffered the loss of a sister, but she herself is a breast cancer survivor. Right after my initial diagnosis, I phoned Nancy after speaking with my father. She introduced to me another key Komen leader at the time, Susan Braun, and together these women gave me words of encouragement and offered to help me put together my medical team. I will always be grateful for their generosity and compassion. They instilled in me an emotional road map to follow: the mountain will be scaled step by step, but I would one day stand on its crest and never look back on today.

Now, two weeks after my diagnosis, with the press beating its drum, I once again reached out to Nancy Brinker, this time with my team in the room. Susan Carter, Komen's director of communications and Nancy's right hand, joined the call. I told them what was happening and that I needed their guidance in how best to handle it. They listened and told me I had no obligation to be public and that I must do what was best for me and think of no one else at this point. I must do what my heart instructed me to do. They and my team all agreed that I needed to think hard about what Soraya the human being, not Soraya the public figure, needed. Whatever my decision, they would support me.

I decided not to be passive. I needed peace of mind in order to go forward, and I knew this rumor would spiral out of control. I did not want that negative energy around me. So I called over the heads of my record company and told them I had cancer. I asked my manager to book a particular cameraman whom I knew and ask him to come to my home. I looked straight into the camera and said that I had been diagnosed with breast cancer and that I needed to step away from my career for a while in order to get better. I asked for people's prayers and for their support in finding a cure for this disease.

In addition to this videotape shoot, the head of the record company wrote a brief press release. My manager and publicist sent the messages out, and that was that. I would stay home for as long as it took. I would close the door to my public life and music career and deal with all of this in the privacy of my own life.

Or so I thought.

Media outlets all over the world picked up the announcement, and my Web site was deluged with e-mails. We received thousands and thousands of e-mails, and they just kept coming and coming.

My assistant helped me read most of them. One by one, it was like a painting being revealed to me section by section. Women who had felt a lump in their breast for years but were terrified of a mammogram wrote to me. Husbands wrote of their wives not wanting to leave the house because they felt ugly without their hair. Other women shared how they had opted out of a treatment for fear of losing their breasts and their hair because they were sure their partners would leave them. And still others wrote to share their stories of survival with me. Entire churches were praying for me, and young people were writing to say that they had volunteered at a charity event or had run at a Race for the Cure in my honor. And countless others were thanking me for sharing my diagnosis. But the majority of e-mails were from Latin American women and families sharing their fears and lack of information about this disease.

Little did I know that no other Latina celebrity had been this open before, especially not with breast cancer. It is a culture where the woman takes such intense care of her family that there is no time left to take care of herself. It is a culture where many believe "God's will" is strong enough to render all preventive measures futile, and where negative perceptions of proven cancer prevention strategies dominate. And it is a culture where women roam beaches putting the female form and its assets on display, but at home, where more traditional gender roles, religiosity, and motherhood take hold, talk of breasts is uncomfortable and avoided.

These are generalizations, but taken broadly, it's easy to understand why this is a culture that has traditionally swept breast cancer under the rug. Especially in the Latin entertainment industry, to reveal such a reality would be to expose oneself as damaged goods. Just turn on the Spanish-language channels, watch the music videos, the variety shows, and the *telenovelas*. Flip through the glossy magazines, and you will see why so many of us have trepidations about doing a self-exam that might lead to a cancer diagnosis. A breast self-exam should be a tool for early detection, which would minimize the harshness of the treatment and might even permit the doctors to cure the woman. But because of the lack of information, the lack of public service announcements, the lack of government programs, and many cultural differences, many Hispanic women do not know that most breast conditions are benign (noncancerous), that most breast cancers are not fatal, and that not every cancer is treated the same way. Just as my mom and I did not know a single breast cancer survivor, many women out there—particularly Hispanic women—still equate this diagnosis with death.

As the torrent of media coverage rained down, people were identifying with me in a new way, seeing me in a different light. I was taken aback by this response. My manager's phone was ringing off the hook with interview requests from the United States all the way south to Argentina.

I decided to again pull my team together, and I shared my thoughts with them. I was due to begin my first chemotherapy treatment that week, and the journey would surely be long and difficult. At this point, there was no finish line established, no end point in sight. I needed to be strong and stay focused throughout the entire ordeal. That was never in question. But I felt that something else was happening around me. I felt that something bigger than me or my illness was pulling and manipulating the strings above my head. I needed to listen.

I announced to my team that we would turn down all interview requests. But soon after that, I found myself ready spiritually, physically, and emotionally, and I decided we would hand-select three interviews to do. One would be print, another radio, and the third television, both English and Spanish. But I wanted some rules. As long as the media were going to shine the spotlight on me, I was going to make sure they aimed that same light into the dark corners of the breast cancer issue. I was confident I could have my way because they all wanted to be the first to get me on camera. Nothing attracts more ratings than a painful human experience.

My manager carefully narrowed it down, and we chose the three. Before they could interview me, I insisted they do their homework. Each story needed to include accurate, up-to-date information about breast cancer detection and treatments. They needed to provide relevant statistics to alert the community to the severity of the problem. The reporters needed to make it easy for their listeners, readers, or viewers to access information and help for anything concerning breast cancer, so they needed to research local clinics that provided mammograms, free clinic programs for the uninsured, and provide free preapproved visuals to teach women the correct way to do a self-exam. And finally, the interview's tone was to be positive, informative, and, above all, inspiring. I was committed to terminating any interview if the reporter employed any pathetic attempts to get gratuitous tears out of me. Chances were good that I would shed one or two anyway, since I have always worn my heart on my sleeve, so ambushes were not required.

The interviews were amazing. I met some absolutely terrific reporters. And as I later learned, the coverage they generated was far-reaching. By sharing, I had unwittingly begun recruiting people from all walks of life to join a growing grassroots army of change agents. Suddenly I wasn't just a patient. I was a proud patient advocate.

It is now more than five years later, and I've spent a chunk of my postdiagnosis time as the "Latin Ambassador" for the Susan G. Komen Foundation. I have spoken at countless events in front of patients, doctors, and researchers. I have inaugurated clinics, helped organize free mammogram programs, been a guest of honor at countless health fairs, and done public service announcements for Latin American and U.S. audiences. I am the face of Yoplait's "Save Lids to Save Lives" Hispanic outreach. Other major corporations have partnered with me not only in health initiatives but also in empowerment programs. I have worked with foundations in Mexico, Colombia, and other countries on individualized outreach programs.

Since I began that work, governments that previously avoided the subject are illuminating their cities in pink in October and are sponsoring massive public awareness campaigns on self-esteem and early detection. I had a part in Puerto Rico's becoming the 115th affiliate of the Susan G. Komen Breast Cancer Foundation. I have been present at many Komen events, running, walking, singing, speaking, empathizing, and relating. I am grateful to have walked alongside the first lady of Costa Rica in their first walk for breast cancer. I have worked with the American Cancer Society, Living Beyond Breast Cancer, Y-Me, Las Comadres, Livingwithit.org, and many other groups here in the United States and in Latin America. The list of efforts and wonderful organizations that I have been honored to support goes on.

Wherever I am, I try to plant seeds of hope, and I share my message through words and through song. But as often happens, those faces looking back at me are the fuel that keeps *me* going.

I feel that the decision to be open about my initial diagnosis was made by a force stronger than me. Remember, I'm the quiet one who in the past was happier to be home alone writing a song rather than out and about chatting people up. In hindsight, I can see now that had I not been open, I would have perpetuated the same silence that plagued my mom and failed generations of women. A lack of awareness meant she did not do self-exams or get regular mammograms. A culture of silence meant she did not have someone to empathize with or learn from.

Going public was not easy. One must take special care to deal with one's own demons privately before exposing them in the public arena; but even beyond that, it is difficult. For every educated journalist I am excited to partner with in delivering these messages, there have been two more that skipped class the day they taught sensitivity and the importance of researching an interview. Some ask questions just to get the tears flowing, and sometimes it hurts. I feel vulnerable and upset at myself for letting them get to me that way.

But for each one of those, important people started coming forward out of the shadows. Television producers and directors, writers, cameramen, and photographers would pull me aside after interviews and say thank you on behalf of their mothers, their wives or girlfriends, sisters and daughters. And on rare occasions, another female Latin celebrity would whisper to me that she too was a survivor. Now others are stepping forward, and it's extremely gratifying to know I helped change the direction of the play.

As a child, I dreamed only of becoming a professional musician. I would never have imagined becoming a successful one, albeit one whose fame was ultimately eclipsed by a group of mutant cells. And yet, I could not be more proud of my accomplishments in the fight against breast cancer. I would love to have gotten here on a different train, a solely musical one. But if this is my track, I'll take it anyway.

Chapter 12

REBORN

After having been my mom's caregiver, it was incredibly difficult to find myself in the role of patient. After all of those times when I could not pull out the words or figure out what to say to her, all the times when I felt painfully helpless and unable to ease her suffering, I now found myself watching my loved ones deal with the same complicated feelings of impotence.

It is an interesting dynamic that I live with now, being a patient interacting with my caregivers after having been a caregiver myself. I was an unwilling patient at first, and I found it very difficult to admit that I needed help. I was even more challenged to accept it. Even when I would be throwing up or in agonizing pain from the mastectomies, I would push myself to get up and get myself a glass of water simply because I didn't want to trouble others. It took months for me to learn to utter the words "I need help." My personal space was immediately invaded by doctors, nurses, therapists, everyone. I struggled to make the transition from being fiercely private to having strangers ask highly personal questions of me. I abhorred having to expose myself physically during a most fragile time, but my loved ones were patient with me. And they were aware of the person I was, so they were vigilant about not intruding on my space. Eventually, I accepted that I had to break down the walls I had built around me. Eventually, I began asking for help without feeling apologetic. To remain intact as a human being, I needed to open up fully to my loved ones. For my survival, to give the professionals the best chance to help me heal, I needed to open up to my medical team as well.

My family gave me more than they will ever know. That first year was very difficult, but they were my legs when I could not walk, they helped me laugh when I could barely smile, and they gave me a reaffirming push when I started to veer off my path. I was reminded that life, my life, all life, has a purpose, and that this was my point of self-discovery. And then there were the basic, essential ways they helped me: I always had homemade food in the kitchen. They read up on cancer, researched treatments with me, and helped me make decisions. They learned how to make themselves a better source of support for me. They drove me to every appointment, and they were there every time I needed anything.

Emotionally, they helped me beyond what mere words can convey. We laughed together, and sometimes we cried. They gave me inspiration when my own supply was running low. There were times when I just felt plain tired of fighting, of feeling so sick, and of dealing with the uncertainty of the treatment itself. But it was during these trying times that my true-life companions rose to the occasion.

It was also during this time that many fell by the wayside. In essence, my cancer was a spring-cleaning of my life and of those in it. For the first time, I appreciated the differences among people's attitudes toward their own lives and how that influenced my own attitude and energy. All those who were dark, ego-driven, negative, and out of touch with their own path were let go. After the shakeout, I felt lighter, freer, and deeply in love with those around me. To this day, they are by my side and have never faltered.

At first I had my blinders on: I knew that I had to get better and that nothing else mattered. Whatever sacrifices I had to make, I would do it if it would protect the miracle that is life. After three months of the first chemotherapy treatment protocol, the tumors responded very well. That was all very inspiring and hopeful. Then it was time for my surgery. How can you prepare for something like that? I had always been very aware of my body, and I had forged a career in an industry where my physical attributes had helped me succeed just as much as my musical talents. And yet, here I was. Sure, I would try to get reconstruction, but that was not guaranteed and would only be like a Band-Aid. I was about to lose a part of my body forever and in a very traumatic way.

I decided that I would have a farewell conversation with my breasts and with that part of myself that was going to be gone forever. The night before the surgery, I took off my clothes and stood in front of the mirror in my bathroom. I started to meditate. I tried to focus my energy on seeing beyond the reflection to the deeper dimension of myself. I tried to begin the process; better yet, to jump-start my brain to comprehend the imminent change. I looked at my breasts and said good-bye. I looked deep into my eyes and began to greet and coax out the woman who was lying dormant inside me. She was secure, strong, and able to be sexual, physical, emotional, spiritual, and intellectual on a much different plane. *I need you now.*

Little by little, I took baby steps toward evolving into a more mature woman and a more open soul. Having been fiercely independent my entire life, this was no easy task. But my new life had a way of pushing me hard toward my critical breaking points. A turning point came when one of my best friends took me to my radiation prep appointment. "Tattoo" marks had to be made on my chest to help guide the technicians to direct the radiation as specifically and as on-target as possible. My friend had seen me bald and gray-skinned because of the chemotherapy, she had seen me flat-chested under my clothes, but now I was taking off my top and lying on the examining table. I was so scared that I asked her to stay with me, but then I realized that she was about to see what was left of my chest. I had only just recovered from the surgery and was still not comfortable with my own reflection in the mirror, and now I felt so exposed. The scars were still quite red and my chest looked so foreign, so unhuman, so *not* part of my body. I was terrified, and I froze when it came time to take off the gown. Then I started to cry. I was in front of the technician, a complete stranger, and in front of one of my dear friends. I thought of my mother standing in her shower.

The technician stepped out to give me a moment, and I finally blurted out to my friend, "I don't want you to see what has happened to me."

To which she replied so calmly and with a smile so pure, "I see you with eyes that have not even noticed how beautiful your face is. I love what I see inside, and that has not changed. I am not afraid. Those scars tell me that you are alive! All that is no longer there would have taken you away from me.

"Let's go," she pressed. "Let's get this over with and get out of here."

I gathered strength from her and continued with the examination. I hesitated, but little by little, my gown came off, and symbolically from that point forward I slowly began to allow myself to unravel. I slowly began to learn that it is not about achievement but rather about intention. It was being revealed to me that part of my healing was learning to open up and permit others to come in and take some of the burden off my shoulders. I needed to accept myself as I was now and not hold on to what I used to be.

In a heartbeat I had to unlearn what I thought I knew. My physical exterior did not matter. I had to fight my ego every step of the way until I beat it down. Once defeated, like a raging forest fire that thins the old majestic trees but allows sunlight to reach deep down to the forest floor, a new seedling was allowed to grow: my inner self, unencumbered by ego and society. I didn't expect to flourish while I needed help with bandages, drainages, and skin burns, but I carried myself as if I was more than I was before. My ability to survive was the best quality I had. It made me proud, and that helped my self-esteem grow, which in turn brought all the disjointed pieces of my new reality together into one cohesive, beautiful, strong, passionate young woman whom I truly admire: me.

I needed someone there to hold me after I got sick because I was usually so weak. I needed someone to get my medicines and make sure that the mental confusion caused by some of them did not keep me from taking them correctly. I needed someone to hold me. I needed to be told I was going to be all right. Letting the important people in my life help me was not only good for them, it also became vital to me.

The biggest hurdle for me to overcome during this time was convincing myself that I was not my mother. I would look in the mirror and see her looking back at me. I would have to shake it off so that the image did not stay with me. "I am *not* my mother. I *will not* be her." And yet there I was, suffering the pain she had endured years earlier. There I was, dealing with those insecurities and uncertainties and fears that I was so ill equipped to understand years earlier. It was all so terrifyingly new and yet so hauntingly familiar.

I would constantly tell myself that eight years had gone by since she had died and that science had made huge strides in the treatment of this disease. And yet there it was, her memory, taunting me almost every step of the way.

After much inner turmoil, finally one day I got angry. Terribly angry. I screamed at the top of my lungs. I allowed myself to say out loud the thoughts I had been holding back in an effort to stay positive and focused on my healing. But I knew I had to do this. I knew I had to open up that box inside of me and let those demons out. That would be the only way I could move on—truly move on. I needed to rid my soul of those feelings and I had to confront my biggest fears once and for all.

I remember screaming and crying giant tears. I was furious at the cancer. I cursed the unfairness of it all. I grieved once again for the loss of my mom, my aunt, and my grandmother. I yelled at it for making them suffer so much. And I shouted out my anger for having to go through it myself. I let out my pain for all the physical suffering I was going through and then I stood up to the biggest fear of all: death. I was thirty-one. I wanted to be a mother. There was so much I still had to feel and experience. This was not how it was supposed to be.

After almost an hour of this spiritual cleansing, my breathing slowed back down and my tears began to dry up. My shirt was drenched by all of the pain that I had just released. My head was throbbing. But I felt reborn.

I lay down for a nap, exhausted by this exercise but renewed, knowing that these dark feelings no longer belonged to me. They were gone now, and I would never allow them back in. From this point forward I never looked back, and my *real* new life began, imperfect, but mine. I knew that I would be fine and that I could handle anything that life might throw my way. I made a conscious decision to be forever grateful. Instead of grieving a loss, I rejoiced in the time I had had to enjoy that person. Instead of questioning why, I accepted my reality as a truth and prayed daily for the wisdom to find the strength and clarity of thought not to lose my way. I can wish that none of this had ever happened, but it would be a wish that gets me nowhere. This did happen, it is happening—the sooner I accepted this, the less resistance I would encounter on my way to healing.

I also redefined what healing meant to me. I was aware of the reality of my diagnosis. Chances were very good that even if the initial treatments worked, the cancer would come back. Healing did not mean "cancer-free." Healing now meant living. As long as I had air in my lungs and I was able to laugh and love, I was healed.

Death was no longer so scary. I focused on the smile on my mother's face as she passed. If it wasn't glorious, she would not have reacted that way. And so what if I never became a mom? There are so many beautiful children in my life. I am a godmother, an aunt, and a best friend to a number of amazing children. My influence on their lives is clear, and their gifts to my life are priceless. It may be the ultimate form of looking on the bright side, but this change of plans in my life could allow me to impact the world in a significant and everlasting way. That became my new plan.

Speaking of plans, that was one of my final hurdles. We can make all of the plans in the world. We can schedule, dream, prepare, organize, and think that we are in control. But in truth, we are not. Life has a rhythm of its own, and it is up to us to stay light on our feet to manage its tidal shifts. Sometimes the diversions are minimal, and other times they shatter everything in their path. But the less I became attached to the idea that I could somehow plan out my days, the more easily I absorbed this new reality.

Through this illness, I discovered the "moment"—the importance of living a life full of life right here and right now. Why wait until tomorrow if we can do it now? The more I pulled away, the more easily events began to flow. New, more inspiring, and more empowering work began finding its way toward me. When I thought that I would have to be home and out of work because of my treatment, opportunities flowed in. I believed in myself. Not in the person I used to be and not in the person I wished to be; I fell in love with who I was.

Little did I know that this life lesson would be so important for me in the future.

Eventually, I healed. I awoke at ten one morning months after the surgery, sat up in bed, and took a deep breath. Only then did I realize that all of my breathing for the last weeks and months had been so shallow. All of my fear, uncertainty, and pain kept my lungs from letting the air in and out as they should. But not that morning. Now I was truly breathing once again. I had developed a habit of taking a self-inventory every morning by asking myself, "How are you?" My answer had usually been "Not so bad." But today my response was "I feel good . . . really good!"

I had turned an important corner. This was the moment I wrote "No One Else," a song I vowed would be used to help other women like me and for which any profits would forever go toward the breast cancer cause.

Still, I had to do everything in my power to regain control over my body. I continued stretching every day, but with more determination. I did so until I resumed full mobility in both of my arms, with no limitations whatsoever. At first I could barely pick up a guitar, and even two years after the surgery I struggled with the movement of strapping on a guitar onstage. But that is a thing of the past. I struggled with a mild case of lymphedema, but I rushed to a therapist at its first sign, learned how to do my own self-massage, learned how to use compression bandages, and now I never get on an airplane without a compression sleeve and glove. My left hand looks exactly like my right.

I am fully able to play the guitar and do whatever else I choose to do.

More than a year after the mastectomies, I was able to get recon-structive surgery. In reality, all that did was make my life simpler in basic ways, like wearing a dress or going to the beach. But that year of being flat-chested pushed me to "grow up." As I healed on the outside, I was growing stronger on the inside. It felt as if new layers of my soul were forming. The more the disease took away from me, the thicker these layers grew. A part of me was gone forever, and in truth I missed it. I missed it sexually, I missed it physically, I missed it just because it was mine and I had to sacrifice it for a greater good. But now that I was feeling better, I somehow, slowly, began to make sense of this senseless reality.

Soon enough, my passion for music met up with my passion for my mission, which was educating Latina women about the importance of awareness and early detection. After writing "No One Else," when the songs started flowing again, they were stronger, reflecting the things going on inside me. I not only had music I wanted to share, but I knew that a marriage between my music and my mission would give me a platform from which I could reach even more women.

By 2003, I had a new record contract and my fourth record was in stores. I hadn't wanted to write a cancer survival record, but of course, that was part of who I was now. The first single was an anthem for sur-vival, and it went to number one in the United States. I was proud of it, but prouder still of all the opportunities it gave me to speak out.

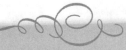

No One Else

It came out of nowhere and shot through my heart
Time stood still as my world fell apart
Four simple words turned me upside down
As my life was spinning, I reached for steady ground

With an army in my soul, soldiers of love, warriors of faith
Fighting a battle against the enemy with no face

I am breathing once again
Time has shown me the power of my strength
This journey is an ever-winding road
And I will walk it proud, tall and strong
And as I'm standing face to face with myself
I thank the Lord I'm no one else

There were days filled with anger, and nights lost in tears
I searched for courage in spite of the fear
In the midst of the madness, I found a quiet space
in simple moments, in a tender embrace

I am breathing once again
Time has shown me the power of my strength
This journey is an ever-winding road
And I will walk it proud, tall and strong
And as I'm standing face to face with myself
I thank the Lord I'm no one else

(continued)

No One Else *(continued)*

In my darkest hour, when I could barely see
I found the essence of a woman I never dreamed I could be

Now, I am breathing once again
Time has shown me the power of my strength
This journey is an ever-winding road
And I will walk it proud, tall and strong
And as I'm standing face to face with myself
And as I'm standing face to face with myself
As I'm standing face to face with myself
I thank the Lord I'm no one else

Lyrics by Soraya. A song written to benefit breast cancer awareness. Copyright ©2001 Yami Music Publishing, Inc. (BMI). All rights reserved.

MEMORIES

From Soraya's first big hit in 1996 through her
diagnosis and comeback in 2003

*S*oraya's first single, "Suddenly"/"De Repente," was released in January 1996 and quickly became a number-one hit in Mexico, Colombia, the United States, Peru, Argentina, Chile, and all of Central America. In the United States, the song was played widely on adult contemporary and pop radio stations. Her second single, "Avalanche," also hit the Top 10. The song dealt with Soraya's own thoughts of the world toppling around her and was inspired by Stevie Nicks's "Landslide," a song Soraya credited with making her a better songwriter.

It was a huge debut for the new artist, and Soraya became an overnight sensation. And yet, the good fortune was bittersweet, as she was still grieving the loss of her mother, to whom she dedicated her first album, titled *On Nights Like This* after the tribute song she had written about dealing with that loss. The song by the same name was also released as a single, and Soraya would later be asked to play it at many breast cancer events.

JOYCE FLEMING
Soraya's personal manager and close friend

I first met Soraya in 1996 as her first hits were breaking. I owned a production company at the time, and I had recently inherited The Studio, a well-known rehearsal venue in Miami for both local and touring musicians. Before me, it was owned and operated by "Mother Mary of Rock and Roll"—who also happened to be my mother by birth, meaning, I practically grew up in the rock and roll business, learning all aspects of it.

I was the first one in to The Studio that day. The buzzer rang, and there was this beautiful girl standing at the front door, holding her guitar. I asked her how she got there and she said, "I drove myself." I said, "Where's your team?" and she said, "That's what I'd like to know." She was very pleasant, but it was obvious that someone was letting her down. As always at The Studio, we would let the artists settle in, and later we would check on them, but mostly we tried to give them their privacy. So I set her up, and then went back to my office, leaving her alone.

Only ten minutes later, the phone rang. It was Soraya's Los Angeles–based management calling. Soraya not only needed to rehearse, but evidently she desperately needed a new tour manager, and they asked if I could do it. Things were happening so fast for her that the team wasn't very organized yet, which is to be expected. But once I got to know her, I understood why everyone was so anxious to pull it together. Soraya was so disciplined and professional, she set a high bar for others to live up to.

That day was the beginning of not only an amazing professional experience, but a ten-year personal relationship that would forever alter my outlook on life.

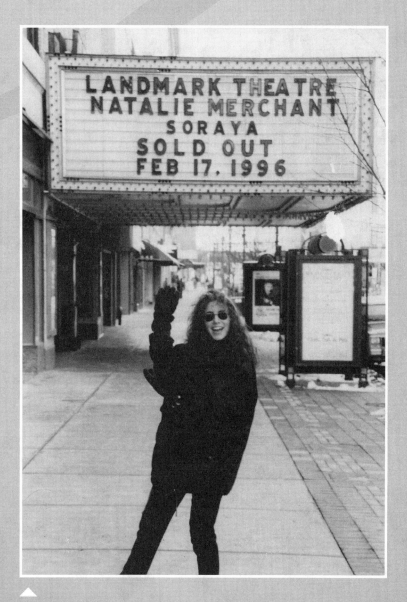

A public figure for barely six weeks, Soraya got a kick out of seeing her name on the marquee along with Natalie Merchant's.

ITZEL DIAZ

Then marketing manager for PolyGram International and later one of Soraya's most trusted musical colleagues and her closest friend

Promoting her first album was a totally new experience for Soraya, and there was no time for learning. She had become a "priority artist" and I was to teach her the ropes. Things were crazy. Press and media interviews were scheduled from 6:00 a.m. (the early morning radio and TV shows) until 11:00 p.m. (the late evening news and shows). There weren't enough hours in a day to keep up with all the requests.

On this one really hectic day, a TV cameraman wanted more than the regular sit-down interview. He got there earlier than his scheduled time, and with the camera rolling from the moment he arrived, he was filming Soraya's actions. He wanted to capture a

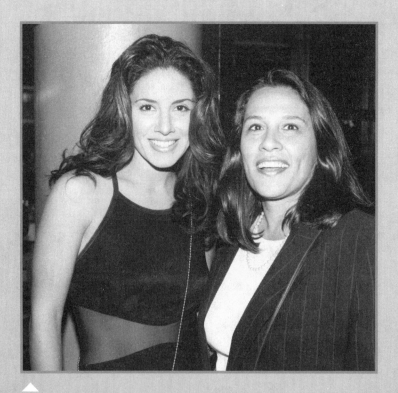

▲
Soraya and Itzel Diaz while promoting the first album in 1996.

glimpse of the person behind the scenes. Needless to say, she was very annoyed. "What is he filming?" she asked me. "Why does he have that camera turned on? Can't you ask him to shut it off? Tell him not to film until we are ready!"

Inexperience, exhaustion, and her wish to be at her best collided, and she locked herself in the bathroom, refusing to come out. Unfortunately, this was one of those times when she may not have liked my response: "This is all part of your career. You are becoming famous, and people want to know about you. If this is not what you want, then let's get on a plane, and we will go right back home to Miami." But she was a pro. She did come out of the bathroom, we successfully completed more than ninety interviews in four days, and—cunning and clever as she was—Soraya quickly learned how to steer each interview in the direction she wanted.

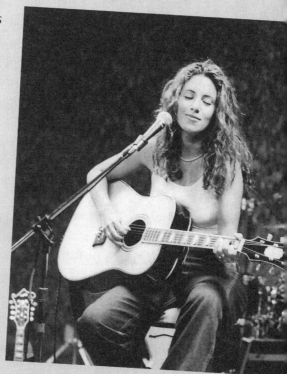

1996. Soraya rehearsing for her first tour.

OLGUI CHIRINO
Soraya's longtime back-up vocalist, keyboard player, and musical director

I was rehearsing in a Miami studio when Joyce Fleming, the owner of The Studio, approached me and asked me how long I was planning on staying in the band I was currently in. I was a keyboard/backing vocalist for a well-known Latin artist. His audience was older, though, and I was in my early twenties. Although I enjoyed playing in the band, I was a bit bored with the style of music that I was performing. Joyce said, "I might have something you'd be interested in. There's a new artist who has just been signed. She's about your age and is the first artist to have two record deals, one in Spanish and one in English."

I immediately thought to myself, Wow! A worldwide market! I was given a CD and I immediately fell in love with the music. I listened to it several times that day and called Joyce to tell her how much I enjoyed the music, the sound, and the singer. She had a style that was unique and special, and I wanted in!

I learned the songs and attended a rehearsal, which was kind of an audition. I remember Soraya walking into the studio and coming over to introduce herself to me. She was wearing a T-shirt, shorts, and sneakers, like she just got out of the gym. She didn't seem Hollywood in any way, but was beautiful nonetheless. She pulled out her guitar and said, "OK, let's see what you got." I remember thinking to myself, "I want this gig; I'm going to shine like never before."

As the first song started, I couldn't help but focus on Soraya's guitar playing—she was amazing! This girl was a mean guitar player. I had been surrounded by musicians all of my life, but I had never met one who had such style, such technique. Then she started singing and I became a bit nervous. As soon as she opened her mouth it was so clear: she was the real thing. Lucky for me, when the rehearsal was over, I was asked to return.

After a couple of weeks of rehearsing, we went out on the road. Soraya was the opening act for Natalie Merchant, Alanis Morissette, Michael Bolton, Sting, and Italian superstar Zucchero, just to name a few. We had a great time. We became close, almost like sisters. We did each other's hair, we gave each other facials, and we borrowed each other's clothes. We talked about guys and our families, and I recall her telling me how she got all A's in school because her family didn't have the means to put her through college and she had no other options but to get grades good enough to earn her a scholarship.

On the bus, from gig to gig, we would sing songs, sometimes changing the lyrics of popular songs to make them funny just for our amusement. I admired the musician in her. She was a classically trained violinist and I was a classically trained pianist, and some of my best memories with her were when she would take out her violin and we would play violin/piano duets. She was extremely talented and a perfectionist. Even when we were just playing around she always insisted that whatever we were playing, whether it be Bach or Elton John, even when it was just for fun, she needed to "feel the magic." Onstage, she brought out the best in me and turned my insecurities into raw courage.

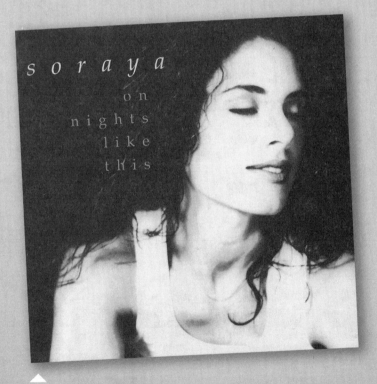

February 6, 1996. With *On Nights Like This/En Esta Noche*, Soraya became the first artist to release twin albums in English and Spanish simultaneously.

As Soraya worked to promote her first album, she was running five miles a day, eating right, and living an incredibly hectic but fun life. With the exception of an occasional Filet-O-Fish from McDonald's and some after-the-show beverages, which at that early stage of her career she sensed were important for entertaining the record company types, Soraya was an extremely healthy young woman.

ADRIANA ARAUJO
Soraya's personal assistant, webmaster, and friend

The day I met Soraya was the day I fell in love with her art. Joyce Fleming was both my mentor and Soraya's tour manager, and she had invited me to see Soraya perform. Guitar in hand, with leather pants and lots of curls, she started to sing the most crystal-clear melodies I had ever heard. She looked and sounded so magical it was hard to believe she was real. Joyce introduced us at the end of the night.

That day—April 17, 1996, the same day her first album was released in Mexico—would change my life in many ways. What I didn't know when we first shook hands backstage in Mexico City was that I was in the presence of one of the people who would most influence my life.

A few months later Soraya invited me to be her personal assistant. Although it meant big change for my life, I was flattered and of course said, "Yes!" For the first time in my life, I left my country of Mexico, and I am forever thankful for all the opportunities this chain of events unfolded for me.

In every place we visited, Soraya was approached by all types of people, all of them fans in one way or another. I observed as she would always take the time to talk to them and to thank them for their time and support. Soraya was an expert traveler with true admiration for the people of the countries she visited, and she taught me to always take the time to admire the culture and to be grateful to the locals for sharing with you their space.

When it came to bracelets, Soraya wore many, and when she traveled, she wore extra. She was never afraid to step into a crowd, and in fact, getting close to people was what she wanted to do. She'd wear extra bracelets just so that when people complimented her, she could take them off and give them away. This wasn't a tactic recommended by a PR firm or something—Soraya was always giving away what she had as a way of creating a bond.

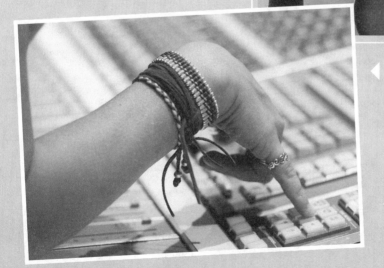

Soraya wearing her Colombian bracelets.

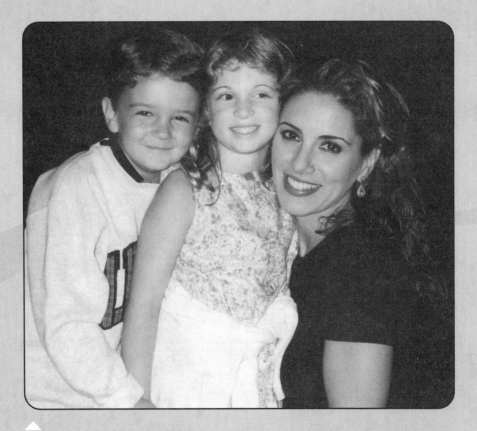

August 1996. Soraya with her nephew Robert and niece Kristen backstage during one of Soraya's American concerts near where they lived. They thought their aunt was super-cool!

JUDY GOLDSTEIN
Soraya's varsity field hockey coach from Point Pleasant High School

Even by this point in her life, Soraya had left a great impression on me. After her first album, when I was teaching health in Point Pleasant, I used her music to help students learn about writing lyrics and how this helps some people deal with loss, relationship problems, and the like. It was such a wonderful opportunity to teach values and the power of the personal choices we make. I talk to my students about making choices for their futures with a Plan A and a Plan B, which is something I learned from Soraya. Soraya always wanted to be a singer, as long as I can remember. She used to bring cassettes to my assistant hockey coach for critiquing. But

118

she was always conscious that she had to have another plan if it was not yet time for Plan A to work out. She worked hard on her dreams and took full responsibility for them—she was never one to expect others to make things happen for her. Now, I show her picture, tell her story, and have my students listen to her music, and then we talk about the songs and what they mean.

Hard work and self-reliance is a lesson I love to teach, and I'm proud that I was able to know Soraya, a shining example of these virtues in action.

*In 1996 and 1997, Soraya's songs exploded internationally and she toured four continents. Worldwide press zoomed in on her deft guitar playing and on the fact that a Latin woman was plucking the strings. In the United States, Latin music was changing as the children of immigrants grew up in a more mainstream music scene and started fusing their parents' sounds and melodies with contemporary rhythms and lyrics. Soraya fit that description, but still, she was a bit ahead of her time. Music writers compared her to Sarah McLachlan and Sheryl Crow, meaning that her music had no telltale Latin music cues like salsa beats and melodramatic ballads. Her fresh sound gave her crossover potential into traditional American pop and rock, but it also meant that she didn't fit neatly into the standard Spanish-language radio station formats in the United States. Still, Soraya's ability to think, write, and interpret beautifully in both English and Spanish put her in a different category of singer-songwriters. Her talent was undeniable.

By early 1997, Soraya was getting critical acclaim. BMI awarded her the Songwriter's Award for "Suddenly"/"De Repente." The same song reached number one on Billboard's Hot Latin Tracks, received MTV Latino's Best Video by Female Artist award, and was awarded Best Pop Ballad by Premios Tu Musica. She was named to the Top 10 Latin Songwriters list by *Billboard* magazine. In the United States, both *Variety* and *Time* called Soraya one of the most influential women in Spanish music.

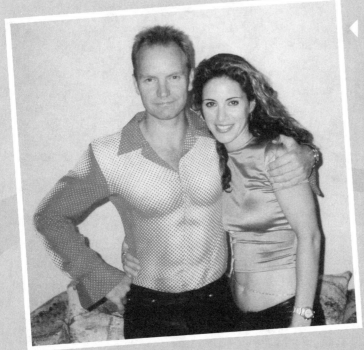

Soraya backstage with Sting, an artist who did many great things for her and whom she deeply admired.

OLGUI CHIRINO
Soraya's longtime back-up vocalist, keyboard player, and musical director

On tour with Sting, Soraya decided to give her show a little tweaking. Among some of the changes Soraya requested, she asked me to play an eight-measure solo in "Stay a While"/"Quedate." Being a classically trained musician, there was never a need for me to improvise, so my skills in that department were nonexistent. I remember talking to her about it and explaining my situation, not to mention that Kenny Kirkland was Sting's keyboard player at the time and I was extremely humbled by his mere presence.

I'll never forget what she told me. She looked at me with the boldest look I'd ever seen and said, "You listen to me. You must believe. Even when you think you're going to fail, change your path and believe. Make it good and keep it consistent, and don't forget to smile." That didn't make my eight-measures moment any better that first time, but at least I didn't choke under the pressure!

*P*romoting twin albums worldwide created logistical challenges for Soraya and her team. As one continent was rolling out the first single from the first album, another continent's team was working the fourth single and saying they were "ready for more product." Like many artists who've faced this challenge, Soraya needed to produce a second album for one part of the world while still performing and promoting her first album in another. For Soraya, producing material for a second album in a very concentrated period of time was to be just one benefit of attending Miles Copeland's castle retreats for songwriters.

GARY BURR
Legendary Nashville songwriter and former lead singer of Pure Prairie League

I think it was the gold chain around her hips that we noticed first. Miles Copeland's castle songwriting retreats were always fun and romantic and wild, but I don't think we expected someone like Soraya. It was only the first night and we were all passing around bottles of local French wine and guitars in the grand dining room in front of a fireplace that was large enough to drive a Hummer through (had one been invented yet).

It was definitely the gold chain. She was swaying to the rhythm of a Latin song, oblivious to the effect it was having on the collection of rock stars, songwriting legends, and hopeful wannabes. Paul Brady, the Irish singer-songwriter, hovered near her, his words, barely recognizable when sober, now just a lilting gush of sounds that managed to sound both poetic and funny. Jack Blades, bass player and singer in the bands Damn Yankees and Night Ranger, with his arms in the air trying to mimic her moves but looking like a marionette being controlled by someone who'd lost half their fingers in a woodshop accident. Both lovely, happily married men with nothing untoward on their minds—just drawn to the beautiful woman with the gold chain.

I was going to take them both down!

She said she was going to teach us all to dance. This was before we knew she sang like an angel. This was before we knew that she wrote some of the most beautiful songs any of us have ever heard. This was before we knew that she could make us laugh so hard we'd beg her to be kind. If it all had stopped at teaching us to dance in the firelight, that would have been enough. She told us the dance was called the Vallenato (Ba-ye-nado). I never could figure out what she said exactly—I think she made up the name. We didn't care. We each took our slightly drunken (Paul might take exception to that—he's never been "slightly" drunk) turns dancing with her. I encouraged my two rivals to "drink up; you'll dance better!" I was trying to clear the playing field for myself.

By the end of the night all four of us had become the best of friends. We would all stay that way for a long time; as long as God let us. I can't speak for her now because I'm not sure what happens when you leave this place, but I know that there isn't a time when Paul and Jack and I get together in any combination, which is not nearly as often as we would like, when that night in France doesn't come up. The dance. The fire. Soraya. The gold chain. Friends found and then lost, but always loved.

PEGGY VAN BEVEREN
A coach, mentor, and friend

As things with her music took shape, things happened so fast. Soraya was making a name for herself and I was catching glimpses along the way. I was prouder than ever! She always managed to send me her latest

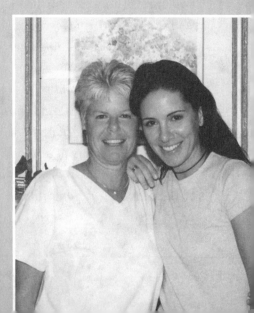

Soraya visits Peggy in New Jersey ▶
while on a break from touring.

CD along with a note, a T-shirt, a poster . . . and I loved to show them off! In phone calls along the way she shared stories about meeting and working with famous singers like Sting and Bon Jovi. She even called to tell me she had sat down with Carole King and written a song together which would be coming out as the title track of her second album. Wow! How cool—Carole King, one of the greatest songwriters of our time, and our Point Pleasant Soraya! I was so proud of her.

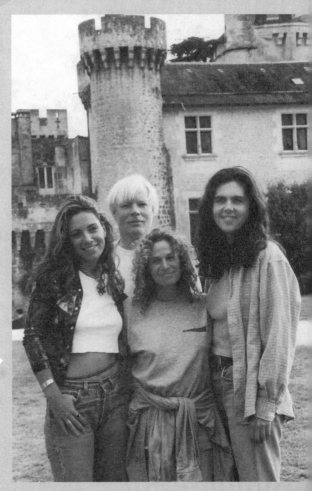

April 1997. Soraya, Miles Copeland, Carole King, and Nashville songwriter Maia Sharp in front of Miles Copeland's castle in France.

ITZEL DIAZ
Then marketing manager for PolyGram International

In the midst of all this craziness, Soraya found a young dog left behind in a laundromat. Forever the humanitarian, she adopted the dog and named her Laundry. She would take that dog every-where. I remember one day we sent a limousine to pick her up for a TV interview in Miami, and Laundry showed up at the studio with her. She sat silently on the floor of the set of a TV morning show while Soraya was being interviewed—on the set! During rehearsals, Laundry would curl up by the mike and wait until Soraya was done singing. Laundry is still alive as I write this today, eleven years old and still running around Soraya's Miami property with two other dogs she adopted over the years.

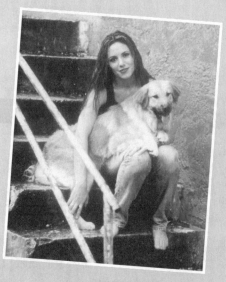

1997. Soraya and her rescued dog, Laundry. ▶

oraya met her idol Carole King at a second songwriting retreat at Copeland's castle. As part of their assignment for the weekend, they wrote the song "Wall of Smiles," the title track for her second album.

◀ Summer 1997. Soraya and Carole King at Abbey Road Studios recording final tracks for "Wall of Smiles."

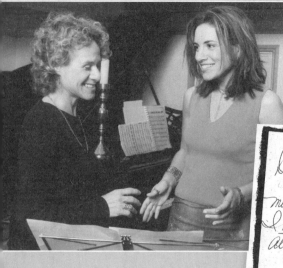

A note from Carole ▶
King to Soraya.

Soraya's second albums were released in October 1997: *Wall of Smiles* in English; *Torre de Marfil* in Spanish. The up-tempo "Paris, Cali, Milan," the emotional ballad "So Far Away," and a few others charted well in various parts of the world.

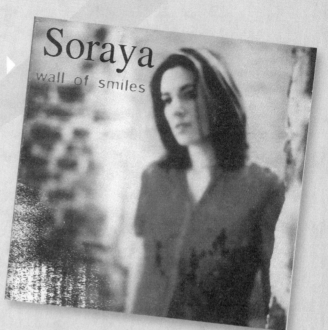

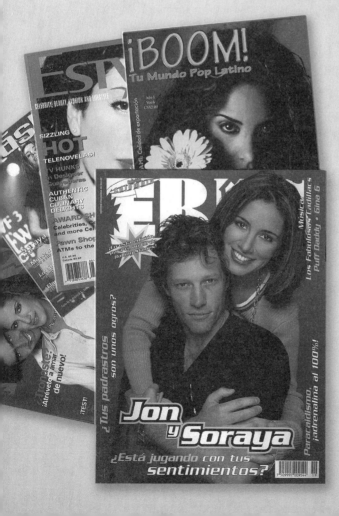

Soraya made the covers of hundreds of magazines all over the world. On top, a Mexican youth magazine features Soraya and Bon Jovi in 1998.

ADRIANA ARAUJO
Soraya's personal assistant, webmaster, and friend

Soraya was very, very funny, and she never took herself too seriously. She had a habit of referring to herself as "Superstaaaar" (but joking, like the Saturday Night Live skit). Whenever a big, pretentious limousine would arrive to pick her up she would roll her eyes, raise her eyebrows, make two peace signs with her fingers, drag them across her brows as if to shape them, then throw her arms out to the sides. In a strong whisper she'd say "Superstaaaar." Then she'd cock her head back to make sure we were all looking at her, laugh at herself, and get in the car.

When she'd be sitting in a chair having her make-up done, she'd turn to you with a dorky smile on her face and you would see that she had placed something black, like a raisin or something, over her tooth to simulate missing a tooth. That wasn't her only tooth gag. She'd stick a square piece of white gum over a tooth and smile to represent having one front tooth significantly larger than the other. Even when she was sick, she was hysterical.

Soraya with Sheryl Crow, whom she met while performing
at a PolyGram Films retreat in April 1998 in Mexico.

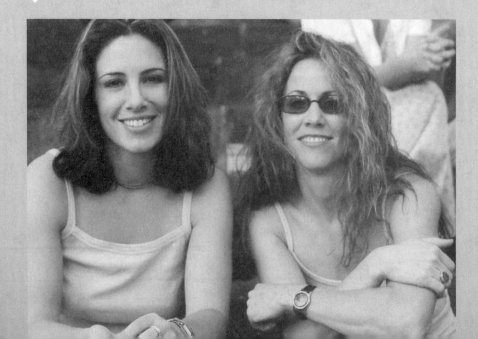

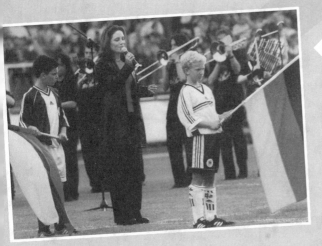

1998. Soraya performing the Colombian and German national anthems.

Soraya was extremely popular in both Germany and Colombia. When the two countries played each other in soccer in 1998, Soraya was scheduled to sing the Colombian national anthem. The night before the game, the German anthem singer became ill, and the promoters asked Soraya if she could fill in. She had already learned some German from spending so much time in Germany, but overnight Soraya had to work hard to memorize the new song. The next day, Soraya sang both national anthems in their original languages, flawlessly.

Early in her career, Soraya had always said that the only thing she ever really wanted from her music was to be able to make a living as a professional musician. After touring heavily for her second album, which came right on top of the first, Soraya slowed down a little in late 1998 and early 1999 to enjoy some simple fruits of those labors. She bought her first home, fixed it up, and started writing songs for her third album.

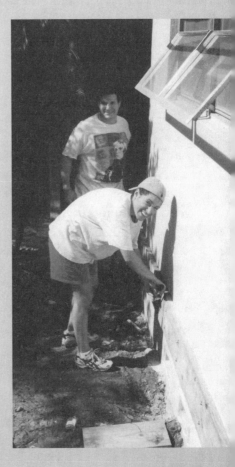

Late 1998. Soraya builds her own deck with help from her friend David.

127

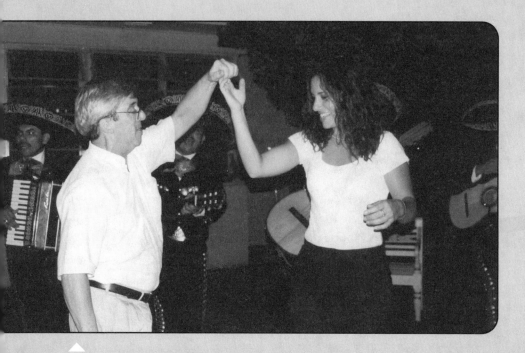

March 11, 1999. Soraya dances with her father, Greg, at her thirtieth birthday party.

*S*oraya loved the hardware store almost as much as she loved music. Ask her what she wanted for her birthday and she'd name a new power tool. By the time she turned thirty in March 1999, she had just finished fixing up her first home. Her father and her record company threw her a party there, out on her new deck. The mariachi band in the background, playing music she loved, was a surprise gift from Joyce.

In the summer of 1999, Soraya turned her attention to writing songs for her third album. That same summer, she met Susan G. Komen Foundation founder Nancy Brinker at a Miami TV fund-raiser for breast cancer, and Joyce Fleming went from being her tour manager to being her day-to-day personal manager working under Miles Copeland.

At the Miami fund-raiser, Soraya had asked Nancy Brinker how she could help the cause and make an impact for Hispanic women, whose breast cancer mortality rates were higher due to the disease not being detected as early. After they met again at Nancy's home, Nancy gave Soraya the role of Latin Ambassador for the Susan G. Komen Breast Cancer Foundation.

*S*oraya's third album was to be another English/Spanish twin release. She had traveled the globe to work with writing partners of wildly diverse backgrounds, and on this record, she was combining her sultry pop rock style with her Colombian and Lebanese roots, and anchoring it all with a heavier "world beat." She felt it was her best work yet, she had a hand in producing it, too, and she wanted to see the record company get behind it strongly.

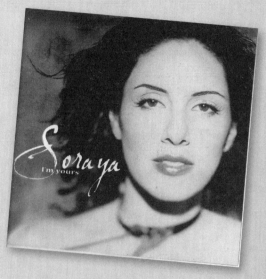

May 26, 2000. Soraya's third album, released only days before her cancer diagnosis. Due to the diagnosis, the English version, *I'm Yours*, was released in Germany only.

SORAYA

Excerpts from a letter Soraya wrote to Manolo Diaz imploring him to promote the album heavily

To Manolo,

Well, my dear, I have finally finished it!! Now that my record is done, I wanted to take the time to write this letter to you.

Either by words, actions, or opportunities presented, you have shown me that you support and believe in my talent and in me. After all, it was you that gave me my first chance, and for that you will always have a special place in my heart.

I have a new sense of urgency, both in my life and in my career. Because of this, many songs were written, thrown away, rewritten, revised again, recorded, re-recorded. . . . I did all of this because . . . I wanted to make my record and be able to say "This is my voice, this is what I want to say."

I have worked hard with my own demons and muses to create something I can proudly stand beside. With your assistance, I have worked with talented songwriters, found a producer that had the strength, patience, and the talent to finally bring my vision to fruition. Without you really knowing it, you have been both a guiding force and a source of strength. . . .

I am swiftly approaching the moment that I will hand over my work to you and your company. As in the past, you can count on my dedication and full commitment to the opportunities you will give me and know that you will find no harder working artist!

We have many things on our side this time. . . . Manolo, I have a gut feeling that we will do something great with this. I know my record will be an impressive calling card for your company and on a personal level, I'm proud—and that's plenty for me. Thank you again for everything you have done for me. You have been a strong presence in my life and I hope a lasting one!

Te quiero,

Shortly after the record was released, on May 26, 2000, Soraya made a quick trip to Colombia to say goodbye to her beloved aunt America, a smart, aggressive businesswoman who had been a role model for Soraya all her life. By June 2000, America was in the late stages of breast cancer.

*D*uring that three-day trip, the moment came that would alter Soraya's life irrevocably: Soraya found a lump under her arm while she was in the shower. Back in Miami the following Monday, June 5, 2000, Soraya was diagnosed with aggressive Stage Three breast cancer. She was thirty-one. By June 19, Soraya's *tia* would tragically succumb to the disease.

JOYCE FLEMING
Now Soraya's day-to-day manager working under Miles Copeland

Only four days after her diagnosis, Soraya was scheduled to appear in New York City at South Street Seaport to perform a concert to promote her brand-new album. Between the emotional turmoil and the Internet research she was doing, she was not focused at all on music. She had been crying for days. But unless we were all ready to go public with the news, she couldn't cancel the appearance. There was never a moment when Soraya considered hiding her condition, but her sole focus was to be on saving her own life. So, she had charged us—the people in her management team and her record company—with figuring out how to make the announcement appropriately. But things were moving too fast. We weren't ready. And without a public announcement, we couldn't cancel the show, or else Soraya would become "the star who sometimes doesn't show up." We had no choice. We had to go. So we packed the suitcases and headed to New York. Miles Copeland came from Los Angeles, and Soraya invited Peggy, her high school coach and good friend.

PEGGY VAN BEVEREN
A coach, mentor, and friend

One of my biggest thrills was in June of 2000 when Soraya called to tell me she was going to be singing at South Street Seaport in New York City, and she asked me if I could come to see her. I jumped at the chance. Once we got there, my partner Sandy and I watched her rehearse. She looked and sounded fabulous. We went to greet her when she was finished rehearsing.

Before we knew it, we were in a limo with her dear friend Itzel, being whisked away to a hotel where she was staying until her performance. I was reeling with excitement. As we all sat and chatted in her room, Soraya left to go into the bathroom. I didn't think anything of it until Itzel dropped the bomb. Soraya just couldn't bring herself to tell me that she'd found a lump in her breast; her worst fears were coming true. Breast cancer.

As the three of us cried, Soraya came back into the room. We hugged, and tried to be strong for each other, but cried some more. Time ran out, and this strong, courageous young woman got ready to perform. We all went to watch her, on a stage at South Street Seaport, as fans cheered, blissfully ignorant about what was going on. And we sat in stunned silence, uncontrollable thoughts spinning through our heads of what was to come.

Once Soraya was back home in Miami, she called up her stylist and said, "You need to come over and cut my hair. I want to have a little cute haircut going into this. I'd rather it fall out short than fall out long."

OLGUI CHIRINO
Soraya's longtime back-up vocalist, keyboard player, and musical director

When her third album was released, I called her and told her how pleased I was with this production. We hadn't seen each other in a while and she asked me to come over to have dinner and just hang out.

The day I got to her house, I did what I usually did when I got there, like drive up to her gate, ring her bell, and when she would answer, I'd either scream something vulgar into her intercom just to hear what her comeback would be—she had great comebacks—or I would sing a song in Spanish. In English it would be something like: "La Sori is . . . An ugly girl . . . Who cries and pouts . . ." She

would parrot it back to me in the
voice of a teasing six-year-old girl.
And this day was no different. I
drove in, and when she walked over
to me to kiss me hello, I noticed
she had cut her hair extremely
short. I immediately said, "What
did you do with your beautiful
hair?" "It's a long story," she said.

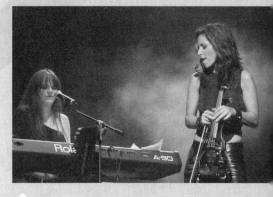

Soraya onstage with Olgui Chirino.

We ate and told stories, and even though we hadn't seen each
other for a long time, it was easy to pick up right where we left off.
Then she said she wanted to talk to me. Out of left field she looked
at me and said, "I have cancer."

We spent a good three seconds in silence just looking at each
other. I started stuttering words that begin with "W": "Wha? Why?
Wo?" Then she explained, "This is why I cut my hair so short. I start
chemotherapy soon and my hair is going to fall out anyway." She
told me she had Stage 3 to borderline Stage 4 breast cancer. I had
no clue what that meant and she explained to me that she was in
trouble. She had already decided on what kind of treatment she was
going to receive and that it was going to be aggressive.

I wanted to cry, I wanted to scream, but I hugged her, I told her
I loved her, and I asked what I could do to help out. She very
sweetly looked at me and said, "I want you around more. I need
you to come here, play the piano, play music with me, and be in
the studio with me to write songs or just make music. I want you to
be here and I want to be productive." Of course I agreed.

So, she started chemotherapy. Her hair fell out. I nicknamed
her Fuzzy. Suddenly this bold, brave, never-miss-a-moment, never-
waste-a-minute girl began to slow down. The chemo affected her
eyesight, and she walked slowly and spoke softly. But one thing
was for sure, her spirit was intact. She was still as stubborn as ever
and she did everything she could to keep her body and mind on the
same page.

ADRIANA ARAUJO
Soraya's personal assistant, webmaster, and friend

At the beginning of 2000 Soraya called and asked me: "Adri, I know you love computers, so I was wondering how good you are with Web sites?" At the time, having a Web site wasn't a common thing. I told her that I didn't know that much about it. Typical of Soraya, always being so prepared, she had bought the domain name "soraya.com" at the beginning of her career. Hiring a company with Web expertise wouldn't be her way. Soraya liked to keep her work "in the family." I learned that day that I was part of that family, and she wanted me to take over this important new project.

A few classes here, a bunch of phone calls there, and with lots of support from Soraya, www.Soraya.com was born, perfectly timed to support the launch of the third album in the spring of 2000. I had gone from personal assistant to webmaster. That first site had warm colors and comfortable textures, but most important, it was a place for Soraya to welcome her visitors with a message that would change as often as her schedule would allow.

The diagnosis came just after we launched the site. I had to wonder immediately, do we put this on there? Soraya's capacity to know the right thing to do saved me from thinking about it. She recorded a short video announcement in her backyard. The team released it worldwide, but also, we published it at Soraya.com.

Only a few short minutes after I posted the video, our in-box started to fill. In the first week, more than six thousand e-mails came in. Some thanked her for talking about her disease. Some were friends or relatives of somebody who had or had had breast cancer reaching out for comfort. Others were from survivors themselves there to cheer her on. And many, many were just regular people who wanted to show their support and send their prayers. I don't think she ever imagined that the Web site would turn the world's energy upside down on her, becoming a vehicle for a true two-way human connection.

JOYCE FLEMING
Soraya's day-to-day manager and close friend

With technology these days, Soraya's video news release had gone around the world moments after we released it. Despite many record company people in the United States who were incredibly supportive of her and were being total humanitarians, scrambling to figure out how to promote a record without its artist, the record company people in Latin America actually called and said things like, "We don't know if we can air this video. . . . This is not something that people talk about here. . . . This will ruin her." If we didn't already understand how deep the cultural stigma was, we found out then.

So we were barely past all these things that seemed like inter- ruptions to Soraya's being able to put down her work and fully focus on her health—the South Street Seaport problem, the pri- vate announcements, the public announcement, those three interviews she chose to give. But finally, ten days into this, we thought we could leave her completely alone. She only had one thing on her mind, and that was fighting for her life. We were to promote this album without the presence of the artist. The first single—released prior to the album—had done well, but they were out of tools. The record company asked, could we please make one more music video? Never in my life have I dreaded a meeting so much as the one where I had to ask Soraya to shoot a music video in the middle of chemo treatments. I didn't want to do it. The music business seemed so trivial all of a sudden. But after discussion with Itzel we thought it might help Soraya to do it. She felt empowered by her short hair, and she was so proud of this record. So we asked her. She refused at first; however, the next day Soraya called me. "Let's go," she said. "OK, I get it" The irony wasn't lost on Soraya that by giving of herself one last time, she was living the theme of her new album—"I'm yours, body and soul" (Cuerpo Y Alma).

A few days later, at a rooftop pool in Miami, in the white hot light of a Florida summer sun, Soraya, dizzy and nauseated from her first chemo treatment, shot the music video to "Where Did You Go?" I'm sure I wasn't the only one there wondering how someone so physically beautiful on the outside could be so desperately ill on the inside. But after that day, we were done with work for a long time. It was time for the fight.

But meanwhile, the record company did something that gave us all a really big idea. Despite the fear of a cultural stigma, the team in Puerto Rico broke new promotional ground by tying the album to a hospital that agreed to give away free mammograms. In Spanish "Where Did You Go?" is most literally translated to "Where Are You?" And they turned that around to mean, where are you, in terms of your health? Using Soraya's music to promote awareness and overcome a stigma—that was a big idea, and Soraya took notice of it. Still, she was going to have to go through a lot before she'd feel strong enough again to decide to make something of that.

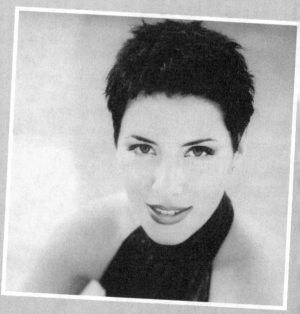

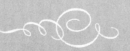 Late June 2000. A still from the last music video Soraya shot before leaving the public eye.

fter weeks of intense chemotherapy, Soraya posted her first message on her Web site since her video announcement of her diagnosis. She had made it a private goal to appear at the Miami Susan G. Komen Race for the Cure in October, and she committed to herself and the world in the posting, "If I have the strength, I have decided I will speak out."

SORAYA
An excerpt from her August 16, 2000, Web posting

In life, everything is possible. Dare to dream, dare to reach for the unreachable. Keep your mind strong, keep your thoughts positive, and most of all, ask God for guidance and help and you will reach your goals. No matter how dark your days may seem, the clouds will pass and life will go on. Often times what we may first think is a punishment or a burden is actually a blessing in disguise. Open your heart and soul and find your way out. The path is aways there, it is just that sometimes it is hidden.

From the bottom of my heart, I thank each and every one of you for your beautiful e-mails. From personal testimonials, to inspirational thoughts, to simple messages of support and hope, I thank you. Along with my doctors, you are all a part of my team and with your help, with God's help, and the support of my family and friends we will win this fight.

Support the fight against cancer. Together we will find the cure.

JOYCE FLEMING
Soraya's day-to-day manager and close friend

By September, Soraya was gearing up to achieve her goal of participating in the Miami Race for the Cure, coming up October 14. She was weak, and she was about to go through a double radical mastectomy, but her goal was pushing her along. She wanted to know if she could use the event as a platform for speaking out. Absolutely! We built a huge press event around it.

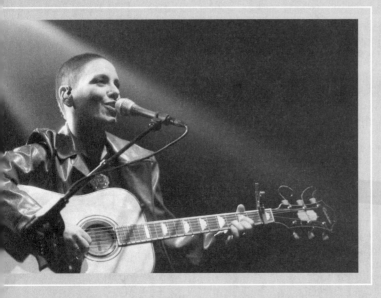

The night before the race, Soraya held a press conference with nearly sixty international journalists. Just three months earlier, she had felt victimized by the press when a sensationalistic reporter tried to get her to cry on camera. Now Soraya was in charge. She had commissioned little hand-made ceramic angels with pink ribbons on them to thank each person for coming, and she hand-wrote a note to each guest, asking them to join her crusade. Before performing, she spoke and answered questions, as did U.S. congresswoman Ileana Ros-Lehtinen, also a survivor. When asked about playing guitar post-op, Soraya gave a radiant smile and said, "I'm faking it pretty darned well!"

The next morning, the local camera crews joined the frenzy. Lolita Ayala, who is like the Walter Cronkite of Mexico, interviewed Soraya as she walked the race. She is a survivor herself, but due to the powerful cultural stigma, had not been able to make much of her condition when it had occurred years earlier. Soraya had personally invited Ms. Ayala to come because she understood the change the highly respected woman could bring about in that country. Nancy Brinker and people from Komen's headquarters also came to lend support. It was a very big day.

TABITHA ALVAREZ SCALIA
Daughter of Soraya's dear friend Rosie, and a friend herself

The morning before the race, Soraya did a radio interview talking about her battle and the importance of early detection. Caller after caller cried to her about their experiences involving breast cancer. It was Soraya's voice that held steady as she comforted stranger after stranger. I cried that morning. It was a strange emotion because a great part of me was thankful—thankful that there were people like her on this earth who could act as a beacon of hope for others despite their own tremendous obstacles. Still in pain from her own surgery, here she was, working passionately to save others from the pains she faced.

Shortly after that race, photos started appearing of Sori with a mystery man by her side. He was with her at the Miami race, and the rumors of romance began. What the press failed to notice, however, was that his eyes were more on others than on her. He is my uncle David, a good friend of Sori's, and it was his job in those days to make sure no one bumped into her. Because under her smiles were the scars of surgery, and she was in great pain.

Something else was going on then, too. She was contemplating what it means to be a woman. What is a woman without breasts? She ultimately answered that question

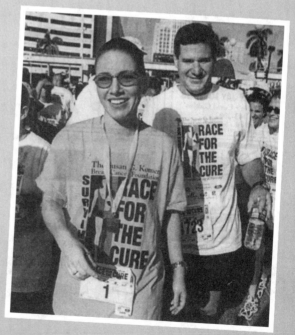

From the *Miami Herald*:
Soraya walking with
mystery man David.

for herself and others. A few days before Sori died, she gave my mother a bracelet, which reads, "I discovered what it means to be a woman." What she discovered is a lesson she left behind for us all: being a woman has less to do with our physical attributes than it does our strength of character.

DAVID CABRERA
Soraya's longtime lead guitarist and session and touring musician

When Soraya became ill, I would always call to check on her while I was touring. About six months after she was diagnosed, sometime in December, I remember getting a call to come over to her house to jam. She was getting the bug to get out there and play again, and so once again, we did a few shows opening for Sting in January 2001. This time it was with the whole band, and it felt so good to see her back in the saddle. But there was something different about her. An urgency. She was determined to champion the cause for women with breast cancer, and it felt like she wanted no time to be wasted.

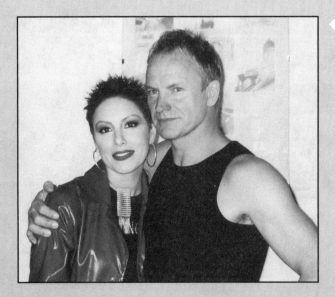

Sting invited Soraya to do five shows in January 2001. It was just the medicine she needed at the time, and she was eternally grateful.

KEVIN R.D.
Soraya's nephew

My tia Sori was a great soccer player! She started kicking the ball around with me when I was real little. When I was four years old she took me to the YMCA and signed me up to play soccer. She started coaching me at home and came to every game when she was in town. She always helped the coach and ran up the sideline telling the other kids how to kick the ball better. The next year, she was home and not traveling, so I asked her to coach my team. We went to the Y and she registered. She was the only woman coach and I thought that a lot of the boys would not want her to be the coach, but I was wrong. We had more kids than any other team, and more boys than girls. We were the Sharks!

Then the season started and we started off a little bad. Sori spoke to all the parents and asked them if we could practice a couple of extra times a week doing drills and learning how to score

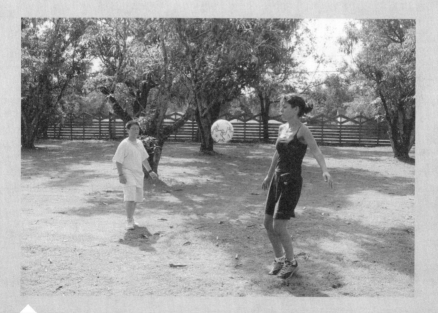

Soraya practicing soccer with her nephew Kevin in 2002, after her reconstructive surgery.

goals. She then became Super Sori. From that day on we didn't lose a single game, and we made it to the championship game. Sori did not care how good anyone played, she always said it was a game and we had to have fun! Everyone played. Not many people knew that she was a famous singer—that was the other Sori. To me she was "my Sori." She was funny, always teaching me stuff and giving me "pispirispis" (tickling me with her eyelashes). But if I did something wrong I was in trouble. Like when I got a C in my music class when I was in fifth grade. She helped me with my projects and still the next report card I got another C. This time she got mad at the teacher and told me that she was going to speak to her and show her the Grammy she won, so she would know that I was getting professional help with my homework and shouldn't be getting bad grades.

My favorite memory about Sori was when we went to New York

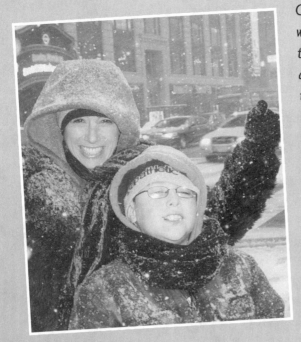

City. She took me everywhere! I told her I wanted to see snow, and the last day she woke me up and told me to look out the window— it was snowing! We got dressed really fast and walked everywhere, making snowballs and throwing them at each other. I miss her a lot.

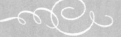

Soraya with her nephew Kevin, whose soccer team she coached in the spring of 2001 while recovering.

JOYCE FLEMING
Soraya's day-to-day manager and close friend

Even after being diagnosed with this rare, aggressive, and advanced form of breast cancer, Soraya amazed those of us around her—she pursued life even more enthusiastically than she had before. After her diagnosis, she says she learned to "enjoy living just for the sake of living." She often shared this thought with us: whether she had five years or fifty left to live, everyone's time is limited, and therefore, happiness is all about finding the right things to do with whatever time you have.

She put her "mission" on top of that list—her work to spread the word about the importance of early breast cancer detection to underserved women. And of course her passion for music returned, and that was how she wanted to spend a great deal of her time, too. And what she was really looking for was a way to combine the two.

*I*n the spring of 2001, Soraya joined Costa Rica's first lady, Lorena Clare de Rodriguez Echeverria, in Costa Rica's first breast cancer walk. As they led the procession down a major thoroughfare, more people joined in at each cross street. This cultural difference was eye-opening for Soraya, and with the sensibilities of a born diplomat, she noted that although everyone is happy to gather at the starting line in the

Soraya walks with Costa Rica's first lady, Lorena Clare de Rodriguez Echeverria, in Costa Rica's first ever cancer walk in March 2001.

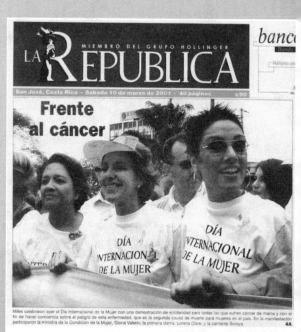

United States, perhaps doing so requires making a public commitment to the breast cancer cause that Latin Americans weren't yet ready for. Maybe in the rest of Latin America, as in Costa Rica, it would work better to allow people to join the race informally as the mood captured them. Soraya found symbolism and poetry in this and spoke about it later: "It doesn't matter whether we all have come from the same place or not; it matters that we finish together." Soraya ended the day by giving a free concert with her band. She had the time of her life, blending mission and music.

ALISON GLANDER PROVOST
Founder/CEO of PowerPact, Soraya's marketing company, and a colleague

Soraya again figured out how to combine these two life priorities—her mission and her music—in June 2001. She wrote a song entitled "No One Else"/"Por Ser Quien Soy," which ultimately became an international anthem and fund-raiser for the breast cancer cause. So that the cause could always receive the profits, she vowed to never include it in her commercial releases.

In 2002 Soraya decided to join hands with corporate America. This is when her team and our team joined forces. Part of our job was to attract choice corporate sponsors whose deeper resources Soraya could tap to reach many more women. One of the first was Procter & Gamble, who generously agreed to fund the "No One Else" music video and Soraya's "Spoken Word" inspirational educational message in two languages for a CD-ROM. After shooting in Puerto Rico, we did promotions in the United States called Prevenir es Querer (Awareness Is Love), in which women buying P&G products got the CD-ROM for free, along with literature on mammograms. The message Soraya was bringing to women's ears was that even though Hispanic traditions may have women putting their families before themselves, in actuality, taking care of your health is the best way to show your family you love them.

Many sponsors and many promotions later, Soraya had distributed more than one million copies of that CD-ROM, surely saving many lives along the way.

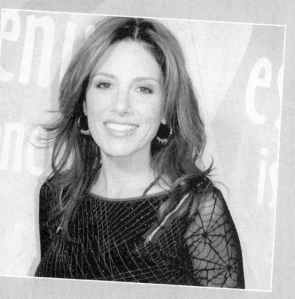

Soraya the spokesperson, at a Procter & Gamble Awareness Is Love event in 2003.

JOYCE FLEMING
Now Soraya's personal manager and close friend

After she recorded "No One Else," Soraya went on to get a new record contract and restart her career. She then released two albums (her fourth and fifth), acclaimed by many to be her best, shot numerous music videos, and performed internationally. She had number-one songs in the United States and Latin America, her music was once again being used as theme songs in telenovelas (Spanish-language soap operas), she wrote songs for other artists, including a hit for Ricky Martin ("It's Alright") and two number-one hits for the Mexican duo Ha*Ash, and she won a Grammy.

But as she mounted her musical comeback, this time we had a whole new set of rules to play by. Her new songs, more than ever before, were filled with themes of survival, hope, and empowerment, and they were the perfect medicine for the crowds she was addressing. This made sense to Soraya. She was one person—a musician who had breast cancer—and she wanted to approach her life in this integrated way. But the stigma was very real, and her new record company didn't always like her methods. It would be easier for them, they thought, to promote a sexy girl with great songs instead of the talented girl with breast cancer. But we were out there, and we were seeing people's reactions. The mission events, the corporate sponsors' pushes—all these things were helping to drive her forward, not just as an inspirational leader, but as a musician, too.

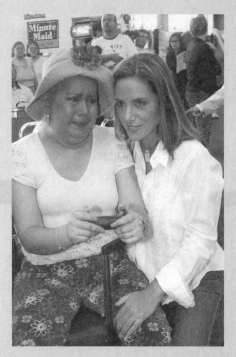

In 2003, Soraya comforts a cancer patient at City of Hope Cancer Research Center in California, and later gives a talk. In 2004, they gave her the prestigious City of Hope award.

ROSE ANN DOMENICI
Managing director at PowerPact, Soraya's marketing company

General Mills's Yoplait brand became Soraya's longest-running and most loyal corporate sponsor. As the relationship was just barely beginning to blossom, Yoplait invited Soraya to perform for all the General Mills employees on their corporate campus in Minneapolis and to attend a breakfast there with the General Mills leadership. Never nervous about meeting anyone, Soraya entered the CEO's office in her charming way and spontaneously proclaimed, "This is my lucky day! It's like déja vu all over again." She told them about getting her big break, about how PolyGram had called and asked her to "bring my guitar and come to an office that looked very much like this. It had a large conference room table. When I entered I was told to take out my guitar and sing, and I had to ask, from where? The top of the table is a fine stage, they said. So, I got on the table and sang," she said. "The table looked just like this table."

With that, General Mills CEO Steve Sanger invited Soraya to perform on his table, which was clearly what she was aiming for. As she climbed up and sat cross-legged on one end, she realized that given the hip-hugging nature of her pants, she was showing a bit more than she cared to. She disarmed the roomful of men in suits when, in a rare moment of normal human insecurity, she said, embarrassed and laughing, "Now, you'll all have to promise me just one thing. No one is allowed to walk around this end of the table." She paused for a beat while they wondered why. "Because these are some very low-cut pants!" The room erupted in laughter.

She was in charge of any room she entered— even when the room belonged to a Fortune

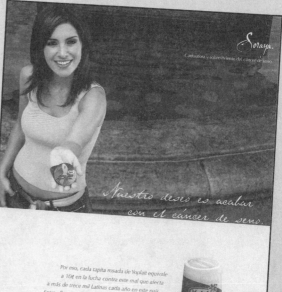

Soraya's ad for Yoplait's Si Se Puede (Yes, We Can) campaign, the Hispanic version of Save Lids to Save Lives.

Soraya speaking to General Mills employees at their Minneapolis headquarters.

500 CEO. And it did turn out to be her lucky day. She forged a meaningful and lasting relationship with General Mills and became a spokesperson for the Yoplait brand and the Hispanic version of the Save Lids to Save Lives campaign, and the two worked very hard together to do incredible good.

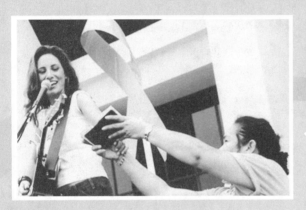

Soraya signs a CD for a survivor-fan while performing for Yoplait at the Susan G. Komen Race for the Cure in Orange County, California, in September 2003.

DAVE CABRERA
Soraya's longtime lead guitarist and friend

After cancer, Soraya's new sense of urgency carried over to her writing as well. Her songs were always meaningful, but now there was even more clarity behind the music and the words. When we recorded "Casi"/"Almost" and the rest of the songs on that fourth album, there was such tremendous spirit and love behind each note we played. Her music created a movement and touched many lives. I remember a young woman coming up and tearfully saying, "Thank you for writing 'Casi.' That song saved my life." I spent eight years with Soraya, and for the first time in my musical life, I felt I was making a difference.

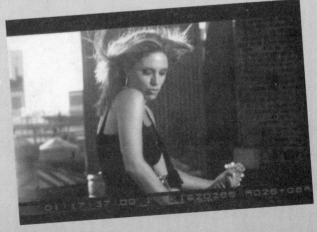

From the "Casi" music video, an anthem of survival on the 2003 comeback album, *Soraya*. The song went to number one in the United States and elsewhere.

Soraya's fourth album, her "comeback" album after cancer, released May 6, 2003.

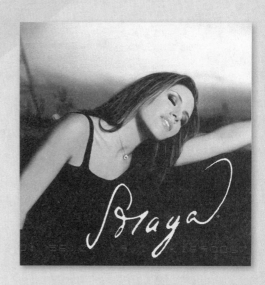

ALISON GLANDER PROVOST
CEO of Soraya's marketing company

Soraya did a ton of press with the comeback album, and she made her interviews work overtime, too. When the magazine Imagen, the Vogue of Puerto Rico, called and asked Soraya to pose in a bikini, she flatly refused. Then she struggled with it for a couple of days and decided that if she could wear a suit with enough coverage to conceal her scars, she could demonstrate to Latina women that breast cancer doesn't take away your sex appeal—your sex appeal comes from how you feel about yourself on the inside.

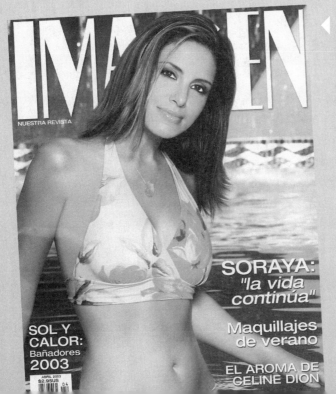

Soraya on the April 2003 cover of a Puerto Rican fashion magazine.

DAVE CABRERA
Soraya's longtime lead guitarist and friend

In early 2004, we were on tour with Enrique Iglesias promoting the Soraya record. At the Buffalo stop there was serious snow, and the kind of cold where all you wanted to do was stay in bed all day. Sori and I were waiting to sound-check outside of the theater. It was dark and snowing, and there was lots of snow on the ground.

We started talking about growing up in the snow, Sori in Jersey, me in New York. We were silent for a moment, then suddenly in Soraya fashion she nailed me in the face with a giant snowball. I

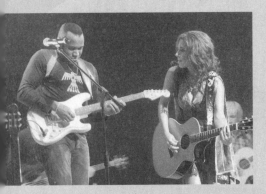

was like, "OK, it is on!" Man, I was chasing her around the tour bus and the cars that were parked there. She kept nailing me—I don't think I ever got her back! We were like little kids, and I don't think I've ever laughed that hard in my life.

Soraya onstage with her good friend Dave, in December 2003.

OLGUI CHIRINO
Soraya's longtime back-up vocalist, keyboard player, and musical director

Besides being a perfectionist, Soraya never wasted a moment of her time. She woke up early every morning and kept a schedule that was so tight, sometimes we would have meetings during bathroom breaks. She kept lists for everything and made sure she'd get whatever the task at hand was right the first time. She would tell me, "Let's take care of it now so we won't have to work twice." On most days she would have interviews in the mornings and sometimes would take me along. She would answer questions, and afterward, whether it was TV or radio, she would take out her guitar and I would take out my little keyboard, and in the same microphone we would do a little "unplugged" set, live on the air. It was real and it was great.

Soraya joins Juanes, one of Latin music's biggest superstars, at his concert in Los Angeles in July 2003.

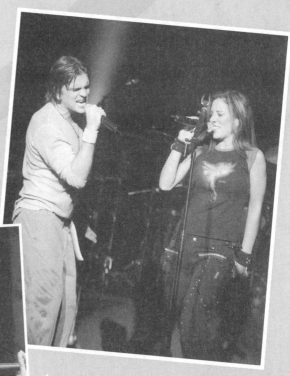

Puerto Rico, December 2003. Soraya does her first full-length headline show since 2000.

Soraya performing in front of an audience of eighteen thousand in Chile in February 2004.

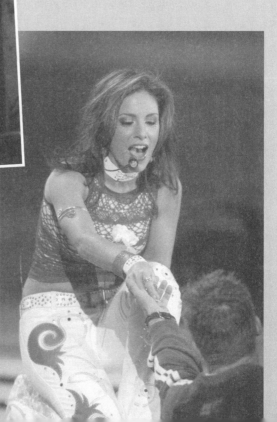

CAROL CROPP
An exec at Soraya's marketing company and a faithful colleague

Each week in Bentonville, Arkansas, where the Wal-Mart headquarters are, about two hundred top Wal-Mart executives come together for a somewhat infamous Saturday morning gathering. In an effort to get Wal-Mart to talk about early detection to its customer base, we secured Soraya a spot to speak at one of those meetings.

As she was led into the room, she was taken aback by the setup of the auditorium. She was to stand in the front of the room so she could address the crowd. However, Wal-Mart's CEO and his team were seated at tables behind her. Soraya wasn't going to be able to address the top brass without turning her back to the larger crowd, and you could see on her face that she was quickly trying to figure out how she was going to deal with the awkwardness of it all.

Moments later, wearing a white leather mini-skirt and white go-go boots (hel-loooo, Bentonville . . .), Soraya walked to the center of the room and faced the crowd. But before she even introduced herself, she twisted backward and said over her shoulder to CEO Lee Scott, "Oh, I see . . . you're going to get the same view of my behind that my band gets every night." The crowd cracked up. Implying that the CEO of Wal-Mart intentionally gave himself a great view could have gone over like a lead balloon, but even in Bentonville, Soraya knew how to get a big laugh.

She went on to tell her story and perform for the Wal-Mart folks. I remember seeing a lot of people in the crowd crying, but I remember being surprised and pleased when I looked at those top executives standing behind her, and they had tears in their eyes, too.

For sanofi-aventis Pharmaceuticals, Soraya became a multi-year spokesperson for a patient support program called "Living With It." As part of her work for them, she created a journal to help cancer patients record their private thoughts. She also made a set of motivational tapes that breast cancer patients could listen to while receiving chemotherapy or walking.

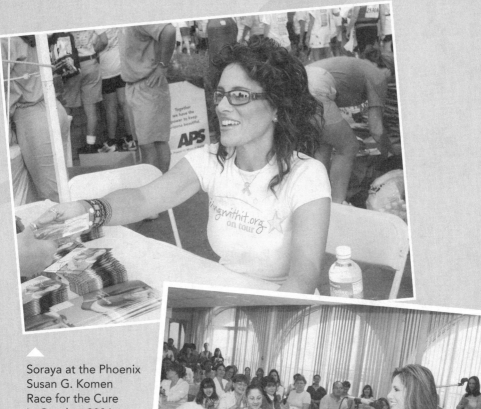

Soraya at the Phoenix
Susan G. Komen
Race for the Cure
in October 2004,
signing journals she
created to help
patients record their
thoughts and
feelings each
day as she did.

Visiting cancer patients in Puerto Rico,
where she performed and gave an inspiring
talk to the crowd.

By the end of 2004, the concerts were once again getting bigger, and the engagements were getting juicier. Soraya looked and sounded better than ever, she had tremendous grace and confidence, and going into 2005, the momentum from the past eighteen months of hard work was palpable.

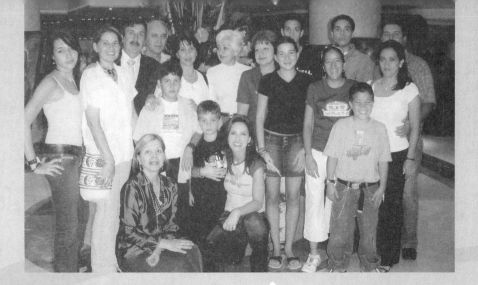

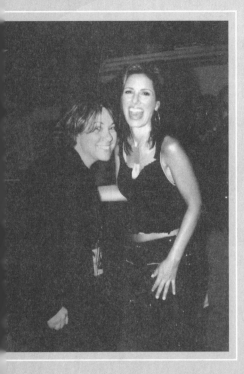

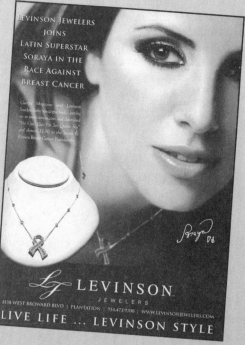

Soraya visits Colombia in late 2004. She has a family reunion and prepares to fill her fifth album with sounds from her Colombian roots.

Soraya and Joyce Fleming backstage in Puerto Rico, 2004.

"The Soraya Ribbon." One of her many marketing coups: a pink ribbon necklace designed by Barry Kronen is produced and sold in multiple sizes by Levinson Jewelers, and thirty percent of sales go to the Miami/Ft. Lauderdale Komen affiliate.

154

ITZEL DIAZ
Soraya's closest friend

Despite all she went through—the lows, setbacks, physically trying circumstances, and sheer pain of fighting her disease— Soraya's fourth album, which she wrote, recorded, and produced, would prove to be her greatest musical triumph, even though it blossomed during a time of intense personal plight. Yet those who knew her well, while awed by her strength, were not surprised by it. She was, in a word, a phenomenon. She had many triumphs after 2000, but the best thing of all came in September 2004: she won a coveted Latin Grammy award for Best Singer-Songwriter for her album Soraya.

We were on our way to the Grammy red carpet, but we got stuck in traffic on the L.A. freeway. I was following the limo in a rental car because we were scheduled to fly back to Miami after the event. There was a hurricane on its way to Florida and we needed to get back and take care of houses, dogs, studio, cars, etc. I had Soraya's cell phone, and it rang about five times in the space of one minute. When I finally answered it, it was Sebastian Krys. "She won," he said, in a very quiet, emotionless voice. "What? Why are you murmuring?" I said. "Where is she?" he

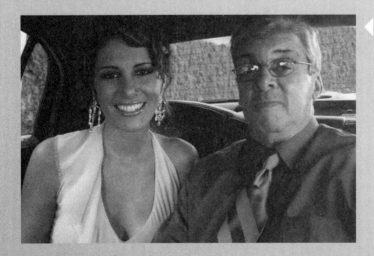

Soraya stuck in traffic on a Los Angeles freeway on the way to the Grammy Awards Celebration with her father, Greg.

Soraya beaming with her new Grammy, in a dress custom-made by famed Colombian fashion designer Silvia Tcherassi—the lowest cut she had dared to wear since her surgery.

wanted to know. "I'm at the event and they just called out her name, and I can't talk too loud. She . . . won. . . . Where . . . is . . . she?" he repeated slowly, under his breath. "She's in the limo in front of me with her dad and Joyce. SHE WON?!" I screamed! And then I started to honk and flash the headlights like crazy. It took them a while, but then Joyce called saying, "What's the matter?" "SHE WON! SHE WON!" was all I kept yelling. When Soraya walked the red carpet, she was beaming and everyone was so happy for her. It was a magical afternoon!

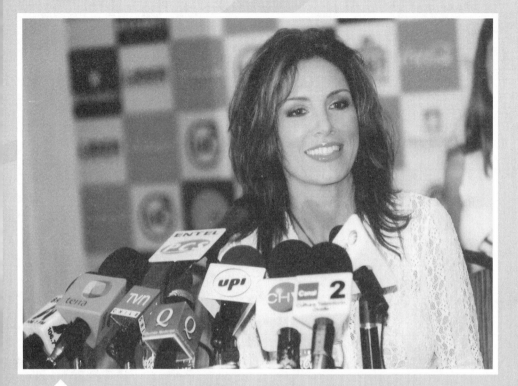

At an international press conference in Chile, after an award-winning performance, Soraya once again mixes music with message. "Turning the camera around to focus it on the disease" was one of many ways Soraya worked to make a difference.

JOYCE FLEMING
Soraya's personal manager and close friend

At the end of each exhausting day, after the races and walks, after the appearances and the speeches, we'd come back to the hotel and Soraya would ask me gently, "Do you think we did a little bit of good out there today, Joyce?" And I'd say, "Yeah, Soraya, I think we did a lot of good out there today."

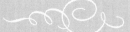

PART THREE

THE RACE

Chapter 13

MIRACLES, LARGE AND SMALL

I was not raised in a religious home. I went to church with my mom, but we did not go every Sunday. Even though I learned about church dogma and memorized prayers, a sense of independent thinking was instilled in me early on. My father taught me not to follow anything blindly. My mother taught me that prayer was my own conversation with God. By not limiting her guidance to the strict confines of the Catholic faith, she gave me a sense of belonging to something much greater and somehow managed to pass on the concept of spirituality in a way that a child could grasp.

The dominance of women in my family also influenced my faith. For my mom, all of my aunts, my uncle, and myself, the biblical figure Mary plays an important role. Maybe she was an archetypal mother figure for all of us, since we shared the common bond of having lost our own mothers. Maybe there was also a cultural influence. In Latin America, Mary holds a much more prominent role in faith at large.

When she was troubled by something, my mom would always turn to Mary for guidance. Later in life I began doing the same. For me there was a familiarity that I found comforting. Even as a child and as a young adult, my prayers were more like meditations, and Mary was my mantra. Since I truly relaxed only when I was alone, that was my most precious time to pray and think. Even as I practiced my guitar or sang a song, and later on when I began to create melodies, I was keenly aware that something greater than me was guiding my fingers along that fret board. I knew I had simply to open my mind and the lyrics and the melody would come forth. I was always very much in tune with my own spirituality. It was something deeply personal and unaffected by outside influences.

In my life, I have been fortunate in many ways. There have been moments that have changed me, and through these incremental changes, I have evolved. I think that all of us have epiphanies, just as I feel that all of us have a creative spirit within. What sets some of us apart is that for whatever reason, when we hear the voice of a hovering epiphany we do not ignore it. We are open to the unexplainable, making it easier to serve as a conduit for these things; to receive the moment in a way that is more than merely fleeting, whether it comes to us in a conversation, a melody, an odd coincidence, a juxtaposition of interesting ideas, or a visual creation. Maybe it's just a way to view some of life's complexities more clearly. Being aware of these things and figuring out what they meant to me was essential to my growth and my understanding of the crises that I would face later on. My epiphanies brought on an escalating evolution in my mind and my soul. I know I could not be writing these words today if I hadn't been open to them.

The first of these notable moments happened the summer after my mom's diagnosis. I was home from school, barely twenty years old, struggling with her illness, feeling powerless to help her and terribly afraid of losing her. I privately doubted the effectiveness of the treatments, and I feared that she was suffering too much. At this point we were still living in Point Pleasant, a beautiful ocean-side town in New Jersey. Being a Pisces, I found solace in the ocean. I would spend many an afternoon walking, breathing in the salty air off the Atlantic, clearing my mind. One gray, breezy afternoon I set out to get some sea air. We had returned from the doctor's office, and my mom was at home resting. I hopped on my bike and set off to the beach. As usual, I took off my shoes, rolled up my jeans, and started walking along the shore, feeling every grain of sand under my feet.

I prayed. I was having my conversation with God. I looked out toward the horizon and asked for compassion, for guidance, and last but not least, a miracle. The compassion was for my family, the guidance was for my young soul trying to maneuver through this part of the journey, and the miracle, well . . . the miracle; there was only one to ask for.

At that very instant, something caught my toe. I glanced down and saw a rusted old necklace. I reached into the moist sand and shallow water to untangle the chain. There, hanging from the chain's salt-worn links was a beautiful metal medallion. I picked it up, wiped off the sand, and froze in my steps as I examined the found treasure. On one side was a classic, orthodox-looking cross; on the other side was an engraving that changed my life.

As I peered at the medal, I saw a trinity of symbols. One was Saint Christopher, the patron saint of the traveler, who offers protection throughout one's journey. According to legend, he helped a troubled child across a stream. The child got heavier and heavier, and the weight almost crushed him. Upon reaching the other side, the child revealed himself as Jesus, and He explained to Christopher that He was so heavy because He bore the weight of the world on himself.

The second symbol was Saint Jude. He is the patron saint of lost causes. His prayer involves asking for help and consolation in times of desperation. Although he was one of the twelve Apostles, there has been confusion between his name and that of the traitor Judas. Therefore, people were slow to turn to him for help. He is believed to have a profound empathy for those who feel that they have been forgotten and left in the shadows.

Finally, the third symbol and central figure of the medallion was that of Mary. There are many "versions" of Mary that my mom taught me. "La Milagrosa" and "La Virgen de Guadalupe" are just two. La Milagrosa was the one on this medallion, and the one that has accompanied me for many years. She stands upright with her arms outstretched and her hands open up to the sky, welcoming and inviting. This

Mary stands for miracles; she gravitates to causes that seem out of reach.

I held that medallion in the palm of my hand as tears started streaming down my cheeks. I just stood there, looked out again into the horizon, and smiled. "Thank you. Thank you. Thank you," I said out loud.

I jumped on my bicycle and sped home. Throwing the bike outside the front door, I bolted straight into my mom's room, where she was lying down. Her eyes were closed, and I had to gently urge her to wake. With tears in my eyes and with complete lack of self-control, I showed her the medallion and recounted my experience to her. Within hours, "Reason to Believe" came flowing forth, note by note, word by word.

I replaced the chain and wore it around my neck for years. That medallion accompanied me until I found someone who needed it more than I did. A few years after my mom died, I met a young woman who was struggling with her own demons and was more lost than anyone I had ever met. Our meeting was brief and quite random, but after talking to her for just a handful of minutes, I reached up and unlatched the chain from around my neck. For a moment, I held the medallion in the palm of my hand and thanked it once more. It had served me well, but now I knew that it had to help someone else. I told this stranger my story of how the medallion had found me and I offered it to her as a sign of solidarity. Maybe if she believed in it as much as I had, she would find some peace in her heart. In as unscripted a way as it had latched onto my life, it moved on to another.

By 2002, two years after I had been diagnosed with cancer, after I had gone through two different cycles of chemotherapy, after I had recovered from the mastectomies, the radiation, and the reconstruction, and as I was on the road to recovery, a mass appeared in my right ovary. My breast cancer was estrogen-positive, meaning that the estrogen being produced naturally in my young body was also fueling the growth of the tumors. Therefore, part of my treatment involved blocking off my estrogen production. Since ovaries produce estrogen, one of the protocols being considered was a hysterectomy. I was opposed to this plan, but when the suspicious mass appeared, my doctors ordered more tests and tried to convince me to change my mind. The gynecological surgeon had even reserved an operating room, as she felt the mass posed an immediate threat to my well-being.

Upon returning from the consultation with the doctor, I went into my favorite room in my house. In this room, all the walls are lined with books. The floor is made of old oak planks, and even the walls behind the bookshelves are lined with wood. I had placed a hypnotic down-filled daybed in that room, which made it quite difficult to read beyond a few chapters without straying off into a warm sleep, although that was often exactly what I needed.

That day I needed to take a moment for myself. The stress of the illness, the challenges of physical recovery, and this new complication were weighing hard upon my psyche. I decided to lie down and do an intense meditation session. I had gotten into the habit of doing a body-length meditation. I would start at my feet and focus on my skin, my tendons, my muscles, my bones, my blood cells. I would focus all my energies on a particular part of my body. I had been doing this for years on a daily basis, and I had progressed to being able to get into full concentration quite rapidly—the part of my body that was the recipient of my directed energy would literally heat up.

As I proceeded through my meditation, I had worked my way up to my midsection. Once I got to this troubled part of my body, I adjusted my thoughts. I called upon my angels (my mom, my aunt, and my grandmother) to help me resolve the questions surrounding this mass. I asked them for guidance and clarity of mind to make the right decision. Then it happened. With my eyes fully closed, deep in meditation but not in sleep, something amazing appeared before me. I felt a pressure around my lower hip/pelvic area. With my eyes still closed, three figures began to reveal themselves in front of me. At first, they were blurry, then they crystallized into perfect focus. As the embrace tightened around me, I "saw" in front of me Saint Jude to my right, Jesus to my left, and La Milagrosa—the same Mary that had been on that medallion with Saint Jude over thirteen years earlier. To my bewilderment, I realized the pressure I felt was the warmth of arms circling me and pressing against my body.

All three had a warm calm in their eyes and a gentle smile as they embraced me hand in hand. I felt no harm could come to me. I was protected. I was taken aback: How could it be? What was I seeing? Was I dreaming? Was this a strange reaction to a medicine I had taken? Then

I let go. My eyes were closed, I was fully into my meditation, and I had never felt such serenity. Then the logical me kicked in, and I thought that since this was such an honor, how could I not engage in a dialogue with them! This might never happen again; I must let this go where it needs to take me! Through my thoughts, I thanked them for being here for me. I thanked Mary for never abandoning me, Saint Jude for keeping watch over my health, and Jesus for teaching me the power of charity and selflessness. I asked them to relieve me of the burdens I was feeling.

This vision remained with me for several minutes. The sensation of feeling their arms, hand in hand with each other and wrapped around my waist, was indescribable and unforgettable. Then as spontaneously as it had begun, the pressure subsided, and my three visitors faded away.

I remained motionless for at least ten more minutes. I stayed focused on that mass and willed it to be gone for good. Then I opened my eyes, without completing my full-body meditation. I could not contain my excitement any longer. I stood up and grabbed a piece of paper. Even though I am not a visual artist—I cannot even draw a good stick figure—I recreated the Mary I had just seen. I wanted to remember her.

The following day, I had a follow-up appointment with the gynecologist. I urged her to do another ultrasound before I made my final decision whether to go with my inner voice or to go ahead with the surgery.

The technician began the exam, and when she approached the area of the suspicious mass, I started smiling. She went around and around the area. She double-checked the notes and the screen and went around and around again. I started giggling aloud.

"What is it?" she asked, slightly flustered by my attitude.

"You can't find it, can you?" I said.

"Actually . . . no. Hold on one minute while I call someone else in here to check."

"Sure, no problem." No problem at all.

I never had the hysterectomy, and my estrogen levels were safely and successfully controlled by other means. The mass was never to appear again.

Reason to Believe

Saw a vision in the middle of the day
Reality slipped a million miles away
As my mind wandered its spirit embraced me
And brought me closer to this reason . . . to believe

Got a handful of burning questions
Living with the burden of good intentions
Having spent years reading in between the lines
Hoping something would stir in my mind

I . . . I've been looking for a reason
And I've . . . been searching for a way
For . . . for a reason to believe
For . . . a way to be set free

I . . . I've been looking for a reason
And I've . . . been searching for a way
For . . . for a reason to believe
For . . . a way to be set free

When I was a girl
And everything was still on my side
The urgencies of certain things
Were tugging at my pride
Now the clock is ticking harder and the years are spinning by
Faster than I should want them to
And I find myself struggling against the same old fears
But through the years I've remained true

(continued)

Reason to Believe *(continued)*

I've been looking for a reason
I've been searching for a way
For a reason to believe
For a way to be set free

I've been looking for a reason
I've been searching for a way
For a reason to believe
For a way to be set free

Chapter 14

SIGNS OF LIFE

I collapsed in my kitchen from the extreme blast of pain I felt in my left hip bone as I walked over to my refrigerator to get a glass of water. The next morning in my oncologist's office, I found out that the cancer had returned. Despite everything we did, despite all the sacrifices, and the amazing new life I had carved out from it all, the cancer had found a way to gather up its strength and come back to invade my body.

Not again.

So began another long journey. It is now my new reality, my new life. A few months after I felt that blast of pain to my hip, the cancer was in my bones and had spread to my lungs and my liver. As quickly as it had sneaked up on me the first time, so it did again.

Now what?

As always, I tried to find a way to keep living, but it was terribly hard this time. I refused to stop. I wanted to keep on working. I wanted to keep on going with my life. Of course, I would have treatment, but

I would dance the dance of a lifetime. Or so I kept telling myself. I stayed so busy—too busy—to really think about what was happening.

This time was very different. "How could it be much tougher than what I had already gone through?" I thought. I could not even imagine what the treatments would be like. Although I knew the odds were high that one day I would be facing this moment, somehow I had held on to the hope that I would never get to this point. But nothing can prepare you, not even your own realistic expectations, and I was left confused, in denial, and completely without my footing. I was frozen. That fighting instinct I experienced in 2000 was not there right away. Had we made a mistake in treatment? Had I done something wrong? Had I worked too hard, traveled too much?

Up until then, I had been doing so well. I had gotten my career back on track. I had released my fourth CD, *Soraya*. The album had won a Grammy, and I had toured many countries. I was living the life of a survivor, and as such, I had found my voice as a cancer advocate. I'd been privileged to be a part of many wonderful programs. Most important, I had found my rhythm as a human being. True happiness had found its way into the depths of my heart.

The shadow of pain that had sporadically shown its face in my life had been absent. I had reconciled with my new body; I had redefined my entire existence. I was more patient and more focused on just being. Through regular meditation I found a way to believe that my life was perfect in its own imperfect way. I am not one of those people who say that cancer is the best thing that ever happened to them. Hell no! *But* the lessons I learned from having to cope with the abundance of emotions were the gift of cancer. My life has been enhanced to the point that even drinking a glass of water is a divine experience. *Simplicity, appreciation,* and *gratitude* are words that I repeat daily.

But with this news in late 2004, I was immobilized; I was overwhelmed with trepidation.

All those doubts were short-lived. I refused to let these feelings of powerlessness take hold of me again. I cried, I screamed, I did whatever it took. I began my reeducation with my doctors and with myself. Plain and simple, I shook myself out of it, as I tend to do. This was not a death sentence. I, of all people, should know that. So why in the world was I acting as if I had no say in these matters?

I decided that this is it now. I couldn't afford to look back. I couldn't look forward. I needed to dig in my heels and get out of this mess here and now and fast. This was my new reality, and I needed yet another new game plan. It needed to be flexible and, most important non-goal-oriented. All I wanted was a good quality of life and the ability to live my life for as long as possible.

I knew I was about to learn even more and move up to an even higher level.

In a very real way, I had become the face of breast cancer in certain communities. I embodied hope and the power to overcome the worst odds. I had shared my story with literally millions of people in many languages, and I know that more than once I had motivated a woman to take care of herself. Now, however, I truly believed that I had something bigger to say, but I was not prepared to say it just then. I could not share this recurrence until I was ready.

I was doing well in my music career, but unfortunately, at least in the Latin market, the breast cancer was considered a liability, and had I revealed that I was fighting it again, I would have been forever labeled damaged goods. There were still those who wished I would stop speaking out so much about being a survivor, for fear that it was somehow hurting my sex appeal and, therefore, record sales. I never stopped.

But now, if I announced a recurrence, the new CD that I had been working so hard on, *El Otro Lado de Mi* (The Better Side of Me), would have been shelved and the book permanently closed on my career. This was to be my fifth CD and the second I would release since the initial diagnosis in 2000 temporarily derailed my career. The songs pouring from my head were my best yet, and I needed to continue working, not just for me, but to prove a point. I wanted to teach the ignorant within the industry that people with cancer can still lead active, productive lives. Sometimes now, because of advances in treatments, you do not even look as if you are under treatment. I was living proof this time. I did promotional tours, and even full two-hour concerts, while in treatment.

I also wanted to be an example for the women in the cancer community and for women at large. I wanted to accomplish certain goals and then reveal that I had done it all while undergoing cancer treatments. I had hoped that that message would give many a little push not to give up and to find a way to keep living their lives amidst the turmoil.

But those were not the main reasons why I did not reveal the recurrence as publicly as I had back in 2000.

Emotionally, I was in too much turmoil. Before speaking out, I always try to work through my private issues first. I find this makes me more genuine when I speak, and it also allows me to be free. I do not write scripts for speeches. I choose to speak from the heart, grabbing my rhythm from the energy of the audience. I am able to do that only once I am liberated from my own insecurities. This time around, I was not there yet. I had to once again deal with my mortality and with quality-of-life issues, yet in a very different and slightly more real way.

Once the cancer approaches this stage, we are no longer holding out for a cure, but simply scratching around for more time. For me it was clear. I had already decided that my choice was not "more time at whatever price." I wanted more time, whatever was meant to be mine, but I needed to be able to feel alive. As long as I was living, truly living, then I would continue on any and all treatment. My doctor warned me that we were now entering uncharted waters. We would try one treatment and hope it worked. If not, then we would find another one. If that one worked, then we would use it until it stopped working, and then we would look for another one. Hopefully, we would not run out of options.

I am now many, many protocols into this treatment cycle, but I'm still here. So far, we have not run out of options. That in itself is a miracle for me, since some of the treatments have worked for only two months at a time. But at least I had those two months. It is a strange psychology to deal with this, but it is the only choice I have. That makes it easier to understand and to accept. When there is no other option, you embrace the one you have with love and appreciation. You learn to relish the moment, be it laughing with a loved one, smelling the aroma of a delicious meal, feeling the warm air caressing your face, or etching every detail of a child's smile in your memory and recording the pitch of his laughter onto your life's sound track.

This revelation was not immediate. It took me months to find this kind of inner peace. I spent many a day and night swaying on and off my path. I touched the outskirts of depression for the first time in my life. I came dangerously close to that black void in the center of my soul that has haunted me my entire life. I cried more tears than I ever thought possible. I screamed, I was short-tempered, and worst of all, I had to deal with something new: constant pain and discomfort. Unfortunately, the cancer was quite spread out, so the pain was everywhere. This time I really felt ill. My liver was enlarged, causing pressure throughout my stomach area, and indescribable pain came from within the center of my bones. I was losing my hair again, I was scared, and I was so close to losing my way.

In late 2005, I decided to step away from all I had known: my music career, my public speaking, everything. *El Otro Lado de Mi* had been released, I had been promoting it in the United States and Latin America for a year, two of the songs had done really well on the charts, I had gotten back to doing full-length headline shows—even in high heels—and with that CD I had done what I set out to do: prove you can go on living while dealing with cancer. The year was coming to a close, and I needed time and space to recuperate. I was also very much aware that my time is not endless—I wanted to spend the bulk of it surrounded by my loved ones, not on airplanes and in hotel rooms.

As I was coming to this decision, on an afternoon when I felt as weak as I had ever felt in my entire life, something wonderful and indescribable occurred.

I was still recovering from the last round of a therapy that we had just stopped because it was no longer working. My doctor was turning over every stone to find my next option. I was feeling tired. The bloating in my stomach was cumbersome and a rude introduction to a less-than-fulfilling quality of life for someone as active as I had been.

As I had done in the past, I turned to my loved ones and I turned inward. I meditated and prayed. I have a stunningly beautiful clay

Virgen de Guadalupe in a niche at the end of a hallway in my house. Next to her I always have a lit candle of Saint Jude. Every day, even several times a day, I pass her and say a silent prayer. That afternoon, I went into my bathroom to get ready for bed. As I was washing my face, I glanced up at the mirror. To my dismay, I saw a geometric figure on my left outside shoulder. I looked closer and it was a square. It looked like someone had taken a bleach marker and drawn this shape onto my upper arm. Out of curiosity, I examined my right shoulder. There I saw a perfect circle drawn by the same white "marker." Strange.

Fortunately, friends were there, so I had people to run to and say, *"What in the world?!?"* Four of us gathered around the kitchen table, and it was not long before one of them noticed something happening on my left inside biceps. A circle was being "drawn," as we all watched with our mouths open. Then a few minutes later, a square started to appear on my right inside forearm. I was a little concerned, but I was not frightened. Instead, a deep calm was coming over me.

The next morning I called my doctor's office to ask if this could be a strange side effect from any of the medications I was taking or if there was an odd dermatological condition that might have spurred this body art. The answer was no on both counts.

Now, three months later, the marks are still there. They are starting to fade a bit, but they are still there. Along the way, they have taken on deep meaning for me.

There is a woman, a dear friend of my best friend's mother. She is a clairvoyant who lives in Argentina. Let me stipulate that I am not much of a believer in these types of things, but this woman is an anomaly for me. We have never met, although she knew of me because of my career and the connection with her friend's daughter. Ever since I was first diagnosed, she would have visions of me, and I would hear of these visions through my friend's mother. Many of them clearly resonated with me. There had been moments when I felt particularly down or weak, and during her conversations with my friend's mother and with no knowledge of my emotional or physical state, she would, for example, volunteer that she saw me like a delicate crystal that needed to be protected right at that moment.

After my recurrence and after two different treatment protocols failed, there was a day I felt hope seep out of me like air from a nail-pierced tire. I was lost and depressed and questioning how much more of this I could actually bear. How much more could my body handle? Was it still worth it? I am a fighter, so these were particularly difficult questions that I was working out inside of myself. I had told no one.

That night my best friend's mother and her visionary friend spoke by telephone. With a sense of urgency, the clairvoyant began the conversation saying she had had another vision of me, but this time it was serious. Someone had to intervene, because I was letting go. I was letting go physically and I was letting go emotionally. She explained that I was tired from all the physical pain and suffering and was contemplating just stopping the treatment and letting things be, but she insisted that that path was not mine to follow. She had crawled into the crevices of my soul from thousands of miles away.

One morning soon after, I showed my friend's mother these marks on my skin. She asked permission to mention it to her Argentinean friend. Yes, of course, I responded. In their next conversation my friend's mom described my skin markings but got no real response. They continued speaking of other things until the Argentinean woman abruptly interjected and said she was having a vision like never before.

Afterward, my best friend's mom dialed me right up and told me of the vision. I wanted to hear it for myself, so I called the Argentinian woman and heard the voice of my "clairvoyant angel" for the first time. Just after she said hello, she began describing to me what I was feeling deep inside and what I was feeling physically. I had the call on speaker-phone with two of my dear friends next to me. She just kept talking incessantly until she got to the subject of the markings. Tears were streaming down my cheeks, because she was touching a part of me that I had acknowledged only to myself. My friends were learning, through her, how daunting my inner struggle had become.

In her visions, and by now she had had several, she saw a cacique. A cacique is an old tribal chief. She could not determine where he was from, but he was dark-skinned and seemed almost Eskimo-like. She saw him sitting at the foot of a large stone, hammering circles and squares into the stone. With every strike of his hammer his eyes would light up like shimmering stars. He had been trying to communicate something to me, and since I had been nonresponsive he chose to transpose these stone carvings onto my skin so that I would receive his message. He was aware of my fragile state and how I had been slowly letting go. Through these symbols, which he said represent the unity of the body and of the spirit, he wanted to remind me that I still had much more living to do. He wanted to remind me of the value of my life, the clairvoyant said. Through my own life example, I had helped many, even though I would forever be unaware of who most of these people were. He knew that I had forgotten all of that and that I was now fully consumed by the exhaustion that was slowly but steadily overtaking me. I needed to be strong and patient because this was not my time to go. I was not even getting close to the time.

I needed to believe this and not let go. I needed to somehow find that light deep inside of me and let it guide me out of this pitch-black darkness. In the clairvoyant's vision, she saw that he was desperately trying to tell me that it was not my time yet. He kept repeating that. The symbols were meant to remind me of that and to keep me from letting go. I spent quite a bit of time on the Internet trying to figure out what these symbols meant, and everything I learned reinforced for me that this was a very mystical, yet very real, message.

Now, I glance down at this beautiful body art and just smile. There are things greater than ourselves, and I am grateful that I seem to have so many of them watching over me.

Live a Life Full of Life

I know the time has come
To rebuild all that's come undone
I know there's got be
More than my eyes have let me see

I'm sending a note to myself
That it's up to me and no one else

I want to believe
I can still fly
I won't let life just pass me by
I've given it all
But now is the time
To show some respect to this hero inside
Inside I'm a dreamer
Inside I'm a child
Inside I am worthy
To live a life full of life

Inside my heart and mind
Grows the love I've been able to find
I've survived stumbles and falls
Losing my step but never letting go

I'm leaving a message for me
That it's time to spread my wings

I want to believe
That I can still fly
I won't let life just pass me by

(continued)

Live a Life Full of Life *(continued)*

I've given it all
But now is the time
To show some respect to this hero inside
Inside I'm a dreamer
Inside I'm a child
Inside I am worthy
To live a life full of life

I'm sending a note to myself
That it's up to me and no one else

I want to believe
That I can still fly
I won't let life just pass me by
I've given it all
But now is the time
To show some respect to this hero inside
Inside I'm a dreamer
Inside I'm a child
Inside I am worthy
To live a life full of life

Oh yeah . . .

To live a life full of life

To live a life full of life

Chapter 15

SINGING TO THE ANGELS

Even though staying alive has gotten considerably more complicated, living has gotten simpler by the minute. It's not easy organizing your life around doctors' appointments, treatment schedules, tests, and dealing with side effects. It is not easy trying to find a way to do what you need and want to do in spite of the limitations that hold you back. It's not easy listening to your doctor tell you that another drug has failed to control the cancer. But it has become easy to share a laugh with a friend, to enjoy a delicious meal, to dance, to be held, and to walk barefoot in the grass. This is the most precious time. The time to just be. These are the moments I treasure most.

Hope. That is what makes it bearable and keeps it real. Possibilities. I embrace the possibility that I might recover. I rejoice in the possibility that all that churns inside me will make me a better person than I was just a few minutes ago. There is the possibility that all I have lived, both beautiful and difficult, has been a building block and that nothing and no moment of my time in this world has been in vain.

And hope. Well, what is left if all hope is exhausted? Without hope nothing has a purpose. Even when life is good and happiness and fulfillment are all around, hope is what pushes us to make it last as long as it can last. Hope is what makes us keep going after the perfect balance slips away, leaving us to believe that maybe it will cradle us once again.

As my body gets more and more worn down physically, and my actions get progressively more edited, my thoughts become more vibrant and I seem to understand it all better. The more physical pain I confront, the deeper I must continue to go into myself to find a way to handle it and not just give up. At the same time, the more of my regular activities I can no longer do, the more I seem to find new ones that are just as, or even more, fulfilling. So what if I can't run three miles anymore? I can swim. I can stretch. So what if I can't work out in a gym with weights? I can pick up a baby and hold her in my arms.

But sometimes it is a lot to bear. Tears fall from my tired eyes because I cannot even breathe easily through the pain. I abhor taking pain medication, so sometimes I put up with more pain than I have to. Sometimes I just scream at the top of my lungs. I scream, punch, and make noises that echo the senseless anger that churns inside. I grunt until I find a release for this monster. That feels spectacular. I have always been quiet, and finding that loud voice has been a true breakthrough. With each day, I find a way to release myself more and more from the cumbersome weight of my physical body. At the same time I cling to my inner soul, since that has become my only truth.

Once I am there, I feel no restrictions. It is the ultimate freedom. What is left to be afraid of if you have found your way to what will be your ultimate state? I am now living from within. Others' opinions don't matter. As long as my inner voices are in agreement then all is well. I am no longer who I thought I would be, but daily I am coming closer to being the woman I believe I can be.

Having been an overachiever my entire life, I have had to unlearn and relearn many things, the most important being that life has its own schedule and it is up to us to keep up with it. Goals and achievements are for the most part artificial creations invented to focus our time and energy.

Living for the sheer sake of living is the greatest achievement of all. I am not being naive. Of course, I know that money needs to be earned, but I have seen time and time again that whatever you emit, that energy and that love that you put forth will come back to you. You will become the person you believe you can be, not the one you are supposed to be.

And then I think of them, of course.

Nayibe, Yamila, and America.

Their suffering paved the way for my survival. What doctors can now offer and what they will offer me in the future is exactly what my mom pleaded for years ago. My *tia* sacrificed so I could receive treatments that did not detract from my quality of life. These women did not have the choices I have. They did not have the support I feel every step of the way. No one was there to tell them it would be all right because no one in *their* lives could find the words they needed to hear. No one was able to sit in silence with them, for within this silence these women would have heard their hearts breaking and the faint whispers of their souls guiding them toward what they truly needed in the moment. I have been much more fortunate in so many ways.

For these women, in their honor, I wipe away my tears.

I think of the thousands of survivors I have met who have reminded me of how privileged I have been. I recount their stories, their fears, and their hopes, and I focus on one woman in particular.

She was about sixty years old. After she sat down in the next chemotherapy infusion chair at the oncologist's office, she started a conversation with me.

"You know that I drive here from the Keys?" she asked me.

"No, that must be quite hard for you," I replied. We were in Miami, and it is about a two-hour drive from her home in the Florida Keys.

Silence.

"You know I was given six weeks to live," she declared into the momentary silence between us.

Swallow.

Breathe in.

"I'm so sorry to hear that. I . . . don't . . . I honestly do not know what to say. I'm sorry," I awkwardly replied.

I saw something ignite inside of her as she looked straight into my eyes. She cocked her head back and laughed with a cackle that I can still vividly hear in my head.

"Oh, my dear, that was twenty years ago!"

What?

Exhale.

"Yep, it's everywhere in my body, but they are always coming up with something. The damn thing gets all worked up, then I come in here for a while and they give me some medicine, then it goes back to sleep. Then sure enough it wakes up again. I feel like this chair was made just for me. As long as it takes, you know. As long as they don't give me a blank look, I'll be back here. It's been hard, but I'm not just breathing, I'm alive!" she proclaimed.

She gave me hope. She summed up what I needed to do. Millions of women like her have died, but for some reason she is still very much here.

I will be like her. I believe in the strength of that possibility and I hope that I may live out those odds in my favor.

I visualize all of these women, for they are my inspiration. I try to recapture their voices and then it happens—every time. The pain never goes away, but somehow it blends in. I accept it and then it becomes like background noise on a crowded street: you know it's there but you never really focus on individual conversations or specific sounds. You can go on with your thoughts under the cloud of the clatter.

I visualize the next generation of women, for they too are my inspiration. Let science finish working out all the setbacks with those of us who are battling this disease today. And for all of those who will hear those four words from an oncologist years from now—*You have breast cancer*—let it be less of a dreaded diagnosis. Let it be a mere inconvenience that can be cured or controlled while keeping a woman's essence intact. Let it be treated without blindly chipping away at her body. Let these barbaric amputations become just a lesson to be learned from in medical books as something ridiculous that used to be performed. Let all of these women live a full life without having to look over their shoulders.

And so I get up. I rise again. I will not let it overtake me. For their sake and for my own perseverance I will not give in. Through sheer sweat, through meditation, and through music I will work through it, and damned if I won't come out on the other side. Sometimes, even when I am fatigued beyond explanation, I push myself physically by working in my garden.

I get down on the earth and work with my flowers and vegetables. I am connected. I swim, ride my bike, or power walk all just to shut my body up and show it that I am still in charge! At the same time, I also show myself that I still can. At least, I can still try.

This struggle, however, is relentless. Only briefly do I get a chance to come up for air, and again I must put on my game face and protect that flicker of light within me. And so I hold on tight to those good days (or sometimes even good hours), or wishfully, even good weeks. Of course I wish it could have been different and sometimes I wonder what *that* would have felt like. Maybe I've paid my dues for the next time and maybe it just plain does not matter. It's pointless, so I usually don't stay in that state of mind for long. I return to my life. This is what I've been dealt, and I have no choice but to deal with it.

I often see life as a candle. I have filled my house with candles of all sizes, shapes, colors, and scents. Sometimes a candle emits a mesmerizing scent, but maybe it burns out quickly. Sometimes it may burn for a very long time, but it never seeps into the air in the room. And sometimes the wick never really seems to catch fire. It flickers but never gives out a strong flame. But all of them have one weakness in common. They are at the mercy of the breeze. One swift gust and a candle goes out. Even kept protected, it will eventually extinguish. We are like that as well. I do not know how long my flame will burn, although I have fought with all of my might and with all of my resourcefulness to protect it from the passing winds. A loss of faith, an overwhelming fear, or sheer exhaustion is like an open window inviting in an unwelcome breeze. I quickly have to snap out of it and run to close it shut.

I know that not only do I burn bright, but I seep into the air in the room. My passion for living, feeling, and loving is my scent. My determination is my flame.

The medical information tells me that my future is grim. Barring a miracle, the cancer will continue to spread. Hopefully, treatment will slow it down. If the disease progresses as it should, I will end up being just a whisper of what I once was. Yet I cannot rule out that something amazing is happening to me.

I have already been that bleep in the statistical charts that sends the curve in the other direction. I do not plan for this to change. I do not see why I cannot keep hanging on the way I have for all of this time so far. I don't see why I cannot be the body in which this cancer does not progress as it "should." I don't see why I should stop believing in miracles. Every moment someone somewhere gets an idea to make a better treatment. I have already benefited tremendously and still daydream about my doctor asking me to come in because she has found a way to stop the cancer forever. It is not such a crazy thought and it is my every intention to fulfill that fantasy.

And with each challenge I confront, I move closer and closer to an inexplicable inner peace. What if I master my mind to the point where I can keep fighting against this thing?

I am not trying to see how many years I can keep away the inevitable, but rather I am trying to prove to myself that what my mother taught me and the principles I have always lived by might actually be right. It is not about living the status quo. It is not living by what is expected of you. Had I done that, I would never have succeeded as an artist or had the courage to do half the things I have done. I also would have been dead already.

It truly is about living by who you are and being guided by what you believe you can be. I am strong. I am faulted. I am talented. I am ill. But I believe that I am courageous. I believe that I am beautiful. I believe that as the cancer moves along through my body, another part of me is healing. I believe that I am worthy. I believe that I have much more to give and to live.

As my cacique reminded me, I have done well in this life. I may never know exactly whom I have touched or how many I have helped along the way, but I must have the peace of mind to know that I will leave this world a little bit better than it was before I was born. A hero does not have to be famous, rich, or talented. Heroes, through transparent humility and selfless actions, leave their mark on their children, on their communities, and consequently on this world. We are all capable of being heroes. As long as my lungs let me breathe, my mind gives me the clarity to think, and my heart allows me to love and be loved, nothing else matters. Once that is all taken away, then and only then will I let go.

As I look down on the squares and circles on my arms, I know that it is my time to reap what I have sown. I know deep down inside that this crop of dignity and grace has taken generations to grow. Many hands have tilled this land. It has been fertilized by tears of pain and by tears of joy. After the droughts and floods, the time is right and a calm has been found during the everlasting storm. I am the lucky one who gets to revel in its delicacy. I get to feel the soil under my nails, smell the perfect scent when the crop is cut from its root. I get to hold it warmly in my hands. I get to stand barefoot in the warm soil and bring the crop up to my mouth and bite into everything I am, all I might be, everything they were, and all none of us ever became.

I want to die with my body, this old guitar that has broken strings everywhere. With one busted string, you can still play chords and a melody. With two strings gone, you can still play a tune. With three, well, now you are going to have to fudge quite a bit. Lose any more and you have to get *extremely* creative. However, it is still possible to make beautiful music with even just one string and a busted-up guitar.

My wood is scratched but still pure, and I have memories of greatness accomplished on this instrument. But I know that as soon as my last string breaks, I will lose myself in a universe where there are no broken strings and where, behind my closed eyes, life is as it should be. Inhale. Exhale. Inhale. That breath is my tempo. Listen to how it moves through your lungs and through your throat. That is so beautiful. Here comes a melody, and yes, there they are, the notes and lyrics floating above me, smiling at me as they did years ago when I was a child discovering them.

Maybe I'm dreaming. Maybe I'm not. Life has pushed me down a long and curving road, and now I have both feet on the ground and my *angelitos* above. I think I'll sit down right here and sing a song. I think it should be about hope, dignity, and grace: a mirror of how these women I knew and loved lived their lives. I know I can still sing to them, broken strings and all.

MEMORIES

Late 2004 through May 2006

I've given it all, and now is the time
To show some respect to this hero inside
Inside I'm a dreamer
Inside I'm a child
Inside I am worthy
To live a life full of life.

—*Soraya, "Live a Life Full of Life"*

oraya wrote these lyrics in 2006 near the end of her battle with breast cancer, when she was taking hold of life for every precious second she could squeeze from it and taking pride in the person she had become through her struggle with the disease. She felt the need to follow up "No One Else" with a high-spirited song of triumph; an indication of how fulfilled and happy she was, even in the face of what would turn out to be terminal illness.

It's impossible not to look back and question whether, since her diagnosis, Soraya always understood that her time here would be short. Was a piece of her strength and hope just Soraya putting on the bravest of faces, as her grandmother Nayibe did? Her closest friends say no. Yet, those who knew her could feel Soraya racing—racing to soak it all in, racing to get it all out, racing to move mountains, and, of course, racing for the cure.

Soraya often repeated this mantra in speeches and to reporters: "Life is like a candle. It does not matter how long the candle burns. It matters how bright the flame is and how pleasant the fragrance is that it leaves even after the candle has burned out." Soraya raced to brighten her flame so more women could hear her, so fewer would suffer the consequences of a late-stage breast cancer diagnosis.

That was the legacy Soraya was racing to leave.

SEBASTIAN KRYS

Soraya's co-producer on her fifth and final album, *El Otro Lado De Mi* (The Better Side of Me)

Although I had first met Soraya in 1997 when I was transitioning from serving coffee in the recording studio to actually having a career in music, we didn't work closely together until 2005, when we recorded what would turn out to be her last album. She was vibrant and healthy, or so I thought. We both took our time in making that album, not just because we wanted to get it right, but also because we were enjoying it so much. We'd work for a couple of hours a day, and then just hang out, enjoying each other and the process. We had connected musically in the way you always dream of—no need to talk or explain to each other what to do, we just knew.

After that fifth album came out in March of 2005, and after Joyce broke the news to me that Soraya's cancer had come back, I went to visit Sori at her house. We spent some quiet time together in her garden. I wanted to put my arm around her, but I didn't know what to do. Because she was choosing to keep the news private, I couldn't talk to anybody about it. I told her, "I don't know what to do, I don't know what this information is I'm hearing, I don't know what the implications are or what the prognosis is, so HELP!!!" There she was, battling for her life, and I'm supposed to be there for her, but it was the other way around: Soraya was teaching me how to deal with cancer. Our conversations soon turned to career advice, real estate, financial planning. Through those conversations I got her broader message: a big part of dealing with cancer is that you go on. You just keep on living.

I was stunned to learn that the return of the cancer wasn't new news. It had actually resurfaced months earlier, back when we were tracking drums and bass at the recording studio. How could that be? Soraya hadn't canceled a single day of work. She quietly scheduled her treatments and then would come work with me six to ten hours a day as if nothing was amiss.

Soraya wanted to go through with record promotion for that final album. I was struggling to understand how and why, because it's a grueling thing to do. There are interviews to do during the day and performances to do at night. You can spend six months, a year, or longer on the road. I came to understand how important it was to her to prove it was possible to keep on living when you have cancer. And did she ever!

She did a showcase at the legendary Pawn Shop in Miami, which is an event to treat the press and record company execs to a live preview of the album, and there were just a handful of us in the audience who knew what was going on with her health. After every long high note she sang, we would all look at each other in disbelief, wondering how she was pulling through. But cancer or no cancer, she was amazing. The music was obviously a source of pure joy for her.

JOYCE FLEMING
Soraya's personal manager and close friend

Why Soraya decided to spend a good deal of 2005 on the road is a big question. Many people in her situation would have spent it indulging themselves or cocooning with family. Soraya was self-less about it—she used the time to get her message out, and if you think about it, she really gave away much of her precious time left on earth. She used her music as her platform to speak from, and of course it was such a source of joy anyway, so it all kind of worked together. Before anyone knew the cancer was back, she described her 2005 life pretty much just that way to Billboard's Leila Cobo, the Latin music reporter. Soraya said, "Basically my life is split in three. My music career. My life. And my third part is this [the fight against breast cancer]. It's a full-time job."

*I*n 2004, to prepare for her fifth album, *El Otro Lado de Mi* (The Better Side of Me), Soraya went to Colombia to rediscover her musical roots. What she found was inspiration in more ways than she could have guessed. As she told the *San Antonio Express News* about the trip, "There's the guitar-based music, the storytelling music, the *cumbias*, and more. I went down there just to kind of, not remember, but just to lose myself in that again. And I met some amazing musicians. And I made a friendship with Alma de la Calle."

To fully appreciate Soraya's final musical work, one must understand the story of Alma de la Calle.

SORAYA
A piece Soraya wrote, and never published, about Alma de la Calle

It started just like any other day. I awoke March 8, 2004, thinking that I was just days away from having a birthday. I meditated a bit on how sweet it felt to give thanks for another year of life. I prepared my breakfast and sat down to read the morning paper. My eyes went straight to a headline that read, "From shoe-shiner to award-winning poet." I was drawn to the picture and to the story of the life of Maria Amparo Amaya, otherwise self-named "Alma de la Calle" (Soul of the Street). Her dignity and pride in the face of the injustices in her life should be an example to all. Personally, her life has become a profound inspiration.

Being a singer-songwriter, life itself is my biggest source. This story was an

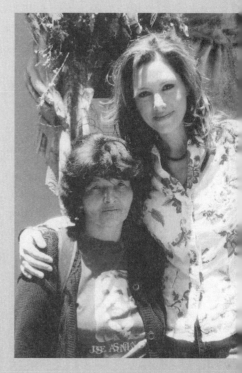

Soraya and Alma de la Calle, during their first meeting in 2004.

inspiration that I could not subdue. But what needed to be created was much more than a song. I went to my writing room, put aside my agenda for the day, and with my guitar in hand I began to write a song dedicated to this woman. I also made a commitment with destiny. If God would grant me the honor, I would one day sit face-to-face with Maria. I wanted to embrace her, to tell her how deep my respect for her was, and I wanted to sing her the song that her courage in life inspired me to write. I personally wanted to tell her that my song "Alma de la Calle" was to be a part of my new CD that I am now preparing, and that with great pride, through this song, I would introduce this beautiful woman to others.

That Friday, I purchased an airline ticket to Bogotá, and Monday I was in a recording studio working on the song. With a little help, I found Gonzalo Guillén, the reporter who brought Maria to my attention. He organized my meeting with her. I have met presidents, ambassadors, and people of great note. But for the first time, I was anxious and a bit nervous when my car was approaching the Institute of Culture. That is where Alma de la Calle was waiting for me. She finally came into sight and my journey began.

After saying hello, she proudly showed me a giant golden key—the old-fashioned kind that opens large, tall doors. It hangs daily, without fail, from her belt. "This is my key to heaven," she told me. I smiled and assured her that the doors are already wide open, waiting for her.

We proceeded to the courtyard where two of her daughters, serendipitously fans of mine, were waiting. We said hello, and the warm hug that followed released a deluge of tears. Her daughter Magaly mentioned that it was her birthday a few days earlier but that today was the best gift she had ever received. Finally, she told me, someone was paying attention to her mother and recognizing the efforts she had put forth her entire life. Antonina, her other daughter, silently took it all in, her tears also releasing years of inner turmoil. In that long embrace I felt the years of pain that these women had endured and shared in their tears.

I began to explain to them why I was there. I showed them the newspaper clipping. Even now I cannot help but smile recalling their expression as they read the article and wondered at the photo! Like old friends, we began to talk in confidence. I told Maria and her daughters that I had brought a gift for them. I got my guitar, pulled out my lyric sheet (which Alma immediately held in her hands and started to devour with her eyes), and, sitting with them on the bench that she normally occupies to shine shoes, I played her my song, her song: "Alma de la Calle."

I humbly sang every word. I had dared to represent this life, this intense life, in four musical minutes. When I finished, Maria roughly wiped her tears and embraced me. Then her daughters did the same. What happened next can only be described by one word: magic. Alma de la Calle began to speak in free form about her theories of life and the Universe. I was mesmerized. She is a fully creative human being, and her mind is in constant movement. She knows more than those whose walls are lined with diplomas. In her tattered lucky blue pants and a T-shirt with Jose Silva's face (the great Colombian poet), and struggling to speak without her bottom dentures, she easily won my faithful affection. She is honest, she is real, she is direct, and she is beautiful. Any other person would have tired in front of so many difficult obstacles. Art and literature have been her saving grace.

Her daughters began reading their mother's poetry to me. An immense love permeated the air. I felt a deep pain in my soul seeing this vision and remembering the story I had read in the paper just a few days earlier.

"Alma de la Calle," Maria, was born fifty-nine years ago into the extreme poverty in which she still lives. Her parents abandoned her and she was taken in by a group of nuns. They in turn gave her away to a woman who cared little for this child, but chose rather to tame her like an animal and teach her only menial tasks. Maria revolted. Her inner spirit led her to hide in closets and read the Bible. That is where she fell in love with the power of language.

She would get punished for not doing her chores, opting rather to devour any piece of literature on which she could get her hands. She soon tired of being treated like a wild animal and escaped into the world of "gamines"—street people. She dressed as a boy to prevent sexual harassment but soon was ostracized by these people as well. She would speak in verse, create stories, and draw on trees, on paper bags. They all thought she was crazy.

Maria began to shine shoes and write poetry. "Alma de la Calle" was born. She started working in and around a university. This way she could be closer to the knowledge that she so desperately craved. However, one night she was gang-raped by three professors and was forced to leave.

Years later, Maria married another shoe-shiner, Eduardo (who I later found out upon meeting him has a little bit of the "craziness" himself!). They have four daughters. Alma taught her daughters to read, and to this day, Magaly and Antonina, the two whom I met, read only their mother's work. They too work on the streets, selling what they can at stoplights and in parks. They are also raising their families with the love of poetry. Amazingly, Alma's oldest daughter is studying to become a nurse.

Eventually, Alma was granted a special permit to be the Exclusive Shoe-Shiner of the Institute of Culture building. She would go there in the morning to earn a few pesos and to be around the world she so loves; then she would move to another building to shine more shoes; and at night she was granted access to a library where she learned to type her poems and thoughts into a computer.

After collecting and organizing her work, she mustered up the courage to ask if she could enroll in a prestigious poetry-writing seminar at the Institute. Not only was she accepted solely on the merit of her poetry, she won a national competition.

And still, she shines shoes. And still, she lives in poverty. And still, she writes.

After sitting with Alma and her daughters for over an hour, she invited me to her home. Without asking where we were to go, I accepted. After a brief car ride I found myself in one of the most dangerous neighborhoods in Bogotá. Honestly, I was calm. I knew that I was in the presence of angels and nothing was going to happen to us. I entered an inquilinato—basically a tenement slum house where there is one shared bathroom and something vaguely resembling a kitchen that is shared by all of the tenants. Upon entering her room I could not believe my eyes. After passing broken floorboards, stagnant smells, leaks, and doorways covered with a mere curtain, I entered a space completely out of place in this environment.

Alma and Eduardo live within four walls neatly covered with her art, and amongst boxes of books and of her writings. In a neatly stacked corner there are cut-off plastic soda containers holding her paintbrushes. Under her bed is a turtle on which they dote, and everywhere there are pictures of her daughters and grandkids. They live in misery but they live proudly. Her daughters eagerly asked me to sing my song for their father. "He must share in this moment," they urged. This time, I could not hold back my tears. The four of them were holding each other as I sang. I was sitting on a metal chair that Alma had painted herself. Then, he returned my song with a serenade of the first song Alma had ever sung for him, and the one he used to sing to his girls every night. They are poor and they have suffered, and yet strong bonds of love keep them together.

Before leaving, Alma pulled out a box full of mini-kites that she has hand-made with the colors of the Colombian flag. She proudly told me she has made one thousand to be given away at her book release party! Her daughters helped hand them out to my family and friends who were with me. Then she turned to me and gave me a mini-replica of her hand-painted shoebox. "Those," she said with a coy smile, "will be raffled off!" Then she reached into one of the many book-filled boxes and pulled out a copy of the two books that were printed years ago. I hugged her with my appreciation but she would not let me have any of the gifts until she carefully and thoughtfully dedicated them to me. The first page of her book, Writing Like Crazy, has this phrase:

"What do shoe-shiners use to give shoes such a lustrous finish? The Essence of a Cloud."

Her dedication to me reads:

For Soraya, I hope you appreciate these street wandering words. Read them alone, in a tenement house, or by the foot of a tree.

—Alma de la Calle

I am back home in Miami and yet I know that my life will never be the same. I have been in the presence of an exceptional human being. As I write these memories, I am glancing constantly at her books on my desk and at one of her paintings, which now hangs on my wall. There are many things in this world that not only can I not understand but cannot accept. The life reality of Alma de la Calle is one of those unacceptable situations. When I asked around Bogotá if anyone had heard of Alma and of her writings, silence was the response I heard. When speaking to her, I realized that she had met many people of great influence in Colombia. She had heard many promises, but most of them never came to fruition. This is difficult to understand. I asked Gonzalo, the reporter, why no one had helped her more. He told me that that is how things are. I urged him to walk away if he would not join me in being part of a change. He stayed.

I made a promise to her daughters that I would make sure that their mother's voice would be heard forever. Before leaving, I asked Alma de la Calle what was her life's dream. This was her response: "I want to publish my writings. I hear that writers get paid when that happens. Then I can buy my own house and build a library filled with books. I want this house to be open for all of the children of the street that have no home, no one. They will be able to celebrate their birthdays here, in the home of Alma de la Calle."

*S*oraya's song about Alma de la Calle is the eighth track on *El Otro Lado de Mi*. It describes Maria's difficult circumstances and her concurrent ability to find beauty in words. In addition to drawing attention to Alma through song, Soraya convinced Colombia's minister of culture to help Alma de la Calle get her work published and to dedicate a library in her name. Soraya and the minister of culture also secured meetings with Colombia's president and first lady, and at those, Soraya focused the cameras not on herself but on the humanitarian issue and the literary jewel the country had under its nose. Soraya then flew Alma de la Calle to be with her in Miami for the release of *El Otro Lado de Mi*, where Alma did a poetry reading at the Pawn Shop showcase.

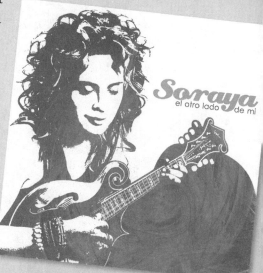

Soraya's fifth album, released in March 2005. Its cover was created by Colombian artist Claudia Calle, and it was nominated for a Latin Grammy for Best Female Pop Vocal Album.

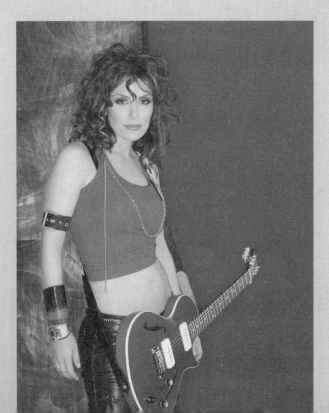

The team went all out for the *El Otro Lado de Mi* publicity shots in early 2005.

JULIET PELAEZ
Soraya's makeup artist and hair stylist from 2003 to 2006

Soraya had a nickname for everyone, but for some reason, it took her weeks to come up with mine. I can recall her bringing it up in every location, like it was weighing on her mind. Then one day she decided to call me "Chompy," a nickname that came from my excessive gum chewing. It was perfect. It stuck.

Soraya would always say "No te lo creas," meaning "Don't you ever believe all this, don't believe the hype." These words always put everything into perspective. One day you have it all and then you don't have it anymore. Things are not forever.

The first single from *El Otro Lado de Mi* was "Llevame"/"Lead Me." Music writers confirmed what her team had thought when they first heard the demo: it has one of the most memorable "hooks" a song can have—it makes you want to sing along, and you just can't get it out of your head. The song became a smash hit in many countries, including Spain, where it spent many weeks at number one on the charts. As Soraya and her team arrived in countries such as Argentina, Spain, and Chile in 2005, people were singing the tune at the top of their lungs while they drove by, confirming that musically, Soraya had ascended to the top once again.

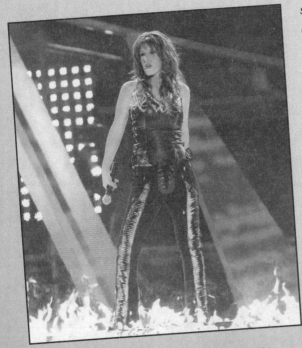

April 2005. Soraya performed "Llevame"/ "Lead Me" live at the Latin Billboard Awards, which was broadcast worldwide.

May 2005. Soraya appearing at the Hollywood Memorial Breast Cancer Center in Florida, with Dr. Sandra Franco (left) and Dr. Alejandra Perez (right).

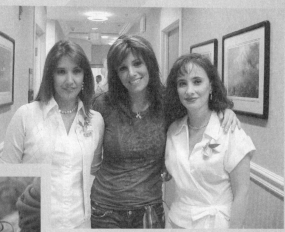

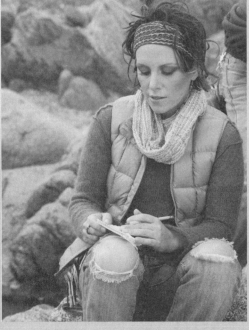

June 2005. Soraya cut her final music video ("Como Seria") on the beach at Islas Negras, Chile, home to famed Chilean poet Pablo Neruda.

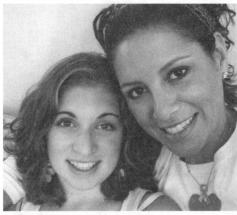

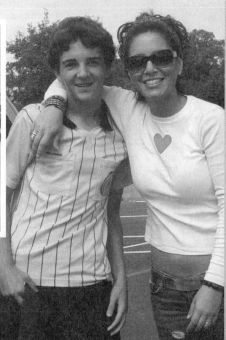

August 2005. Soraya spending time with niece Kristin and nephew Robert.

*I*n 2005, Soraya's star was rising high, and she was booked constantly. She was proud to be able to do this while keeping her cancer in a state of what she described as "controlled remission." In addition to performing two and a half hours at a stretch, Soraya would meet and greet until the very last fan was gone.

At what would unknowingly be her last concert performance, Soraya and two fans had a beautiful and dramatic interaction that stunned Soraya into recognition about what her music had done for others. The fans, a woman and her boyfriend, had been struggling. Something traumatic had happened to the woman and she was suffering from rare, complete memory loss. Backstage, they told Soraya how, in a desperate attempt to revive the woman's memory and rebuild their relationship, the boyfriend had played "Solo Por Ti"/"All For You" for her. It had been the couple's favorite song, and they had many memories attached to it. Hearing the song had not restored the woman's memory, but it had rekindled their relationship just the same. After hearing it, the woman said to her boyfriend, "If that song represents what we had, then I love you now."

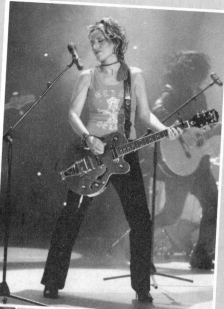

September 2005. Soraya performs in Chile.

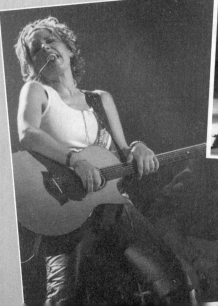

September 2005. Soraya performs in Argentina. She didn't know at the time that it would be her last concert.

*O*ctober is Breast Cancer Awareness Month in the United States and elsewhere, and it was always one of Soraya's busiest months for getting out her messages of awareness and early detection. One of her all-time proudest moments was attending Puerto Rico's first Race for the Cure in October 2005. She had been working with the Susan G. Komen Foundation to make this a reality, and on October 15, five thousand people turned out for that inaugural race—a terrific turnout for a first-time event. At the race, Soraya met Ana Maria Polo, a powerful attorney most famous for being a judge on a popular Hispanic television courtroom show, and an inspirational breast cancer survivor herself. Ana Maria and Soraya inspired each other and the crowd that day.

Soraya crisscrossed the United States in October, appearing, speaking, and performing at numerous races, including the Memphis Race for the Cure, which was to be her last. Despite all she was going through, she didn't complain, instead focusing on what she wanted to accomplish, so she could "look ahead but never down," the line from her huge hit at the time, "Lead Me"/"Llevame."

Soraya revving up the crowd at the Survivors' Celebration at Puerto Rico's first Race for the Cure.

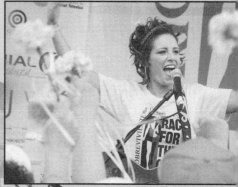

Soraya leading the Survivor March at the Denver Race for the Cure, the United States' largest, with sixty-two thousand walkers and runners.

$\mathcal{S}$oraya's last public appearance was November 3, 2005, at the Latin Grammys in Los Angeles. She was nominated for Best Pop Album by a Female for *El Otro Lado de Mi*. She looked like a beautiful Hollywood starlet that night. The following day, Soraya was scheduled to make an appearance for corporate sponsor sanofi-aventis. Unfortunately, after the awards ceremony, her health took a turn. She returned to Miami, deciding it was time to spend more time with friends and family and to work on this book.

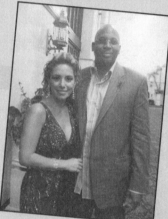

November 2005. Soraya's date for the 2005 Latin Grammys in Los Angeles was best buddy Merle Scott.

Soraya embracing fellow songwriter and previous collaborator Gian Marco, who won the same singer-songwriter award in 2005 that Soraya won in 2004.

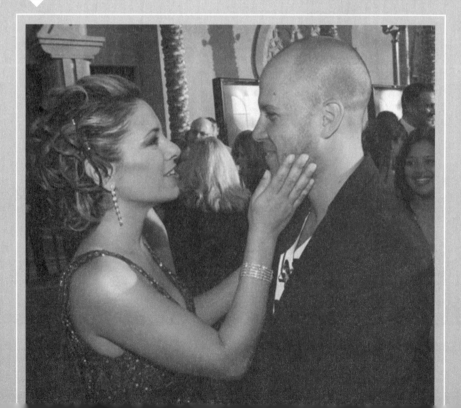

JESSICA CUEVAS
Soraya's cousin and friend

It was late December 2005, and my husband, Bob, and I were headed to Miami to see my cousin Soraya. She was very ill, and we didn't know if her illness was terminal or just another battle to be won. Before our plane had even touched down, Soraya and her friend Itzel had made a plan. One of our four days together would be spent at Shark Valley in Everglades National Park. Knowing our passion for nature and activity, Soraya explained that we could ride a bike trail to view the wildlife and vegetation.

Only later in bed did we whisper our concerns to each other about how Soraya would fare on an extended bike ride. Her discomfort and pain were apparent only from her deliberate movements and need for rest. Not once did she address what she felt physically. Instead she would simply state what she required: "I'm going to sit here for a moment," or "I need an extra pillow on this side of me." If what they were saying were true, this fourteen-mile bike ride would prove a workout to an able-bodied person in decent physical shape. Having visited other national parks, we knew that there would be a shorter, easier loop available to give tourists a sufficient glimpse of the park. We would make it clear from the very beginning that we would be more than satisfied to do that together as a foursome.

We left the house around 8 a.m. and stopped for coffee and rolls at a Cuban stand on our way to the park. Soraya ordered our coffees and the pastries to go in her soft, polite voice. We sipped, shared, and spilled the goodies on the thirty-minute ride, recounting stories about travel mishaps and surprises.

Bob and I waited in line for the bike rental office to open and snagged two rather well-worn, one-speed, manual-brake bikes. Itzel and Soraya had brought their own cycles, but nonetheless a game of musical bikes ensued. Our Latina Goldilocks tested all four within the first forty-five minutes and opted for the cushioned seat of the rental, finally handing her coveted mountain Trek over to Bob.

Pedestrians and bikers crowded the path. Looking at the map, Soraya must have sensed me contemplating the short-loop option. Itzel and Bob looked at Sori. She wasted no time, "Why don't we just head out on the longer road and see how far we get?" Bob quickly added, "There's no rush to do it all today. We can turn around at any time, you know." I knew exactly what she had in mind. I had seen this determination many times before. She was appeasing me with her suggestion of "let's see how far we get." She wanted to go the distance. She had silently asked us to believe that she could.

None of us knew how the trip would end. All we knew is that she needed us to let her at least try. "Everyone have on sun-screen?" she beamed. Bob, a birdwatcher, unassumingly called attention to the anhinga, herons, ospreys, and egrets in the air and camouflaged in trees, uttering their names in greeting. Itzel

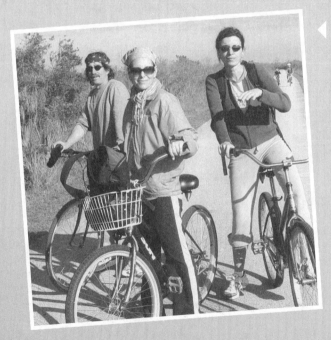

December 2005. Soraya, her cousin Jessica, and Jessica's husband, Bob, on a fourteen-mile bike trek.

and I marveled at the alligators, anywhere from three to eight feet, lounging peacefully on the grassy side of the road or sometimes directly in the middle of the bike path.

We stopped once every half hour to hydrate, snack, lounge, stretch, and take notice of our surroundings. We took turns initiating the breaks, so as not to unnecessarily burden Sori. It was clear that the effort to pedal and the pressure on her body of being on the bike were taking a toll on her. Four trams, one every half hour, had passed us by, and each time I swallowed my instinct to say, "Let's throw our bikes on and hitch a ride back."

We knew the rules. What she needed was to do everything left in her power. What she required was the willingness of others to focus on the possible. We were in. No tram. More Motrin. Double the stops on the way back. Plan the dinner meal aloud.

This was not the first time Soraya had proven herself to be unstoppable. During a visit after her first rounds of chemo, she organized a family get-together at a nearby park. We played a casual game of soccer with family and friends. Weak with nausea, wrapped in a tie-dyed bandana, she craftily stole the ball several times from her soccer-playing cousin and uncle and managed to score a goal. As fate would have it, Soraya's competitive battles would later be fought with herself, testing the limits of her physical, emotional, and spiritual being.

If anyone had timed our bike ride, we would have come in last place. We finished in slightly over four hours. Backpacks empty, souls full. She willed herself every one of those fourteen miles. I savor the memory of my cousin, reclined in the backseat of the truck, exhausted and stiff with pain, her legs propped up comfortably onto Bob's lap, smiling radiantly.

*S*oraya drew a lot of her strength from her faith. She believed in miracles, and here we find evidence of her passionate spiritual life.

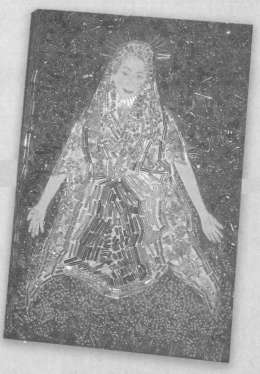

After being taken with La Milagrosa, who spoke to her in a vision, Soraya drew this Mary, then painted her, then beaded her into this Bible cover.

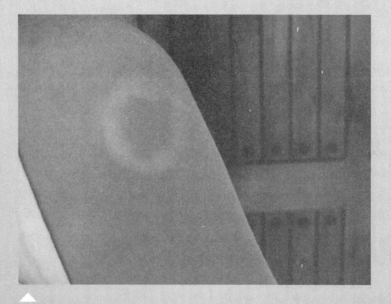

A white circle on Soraya's upper arm, one of a number of circles and squares that mysteriously appeared and remained for months.

By January 2006, Soraya was no longer in the public eye, but the need to express herself through songwriting did not stop, and she wrote three final compositions. In early 2006, she wrote "Live a Life Full of Life" and recorded a demo of it in her home studio. She also wrote and recorded "Face Another Day," a song filled with sentiments of such intense hope and love that it might give others who are struggling the courage and strength to do just what her words urge: face another day.

Face Another Day

Laid my head on your chest tonight
Let your breath be my guide
Up and down thought I was flying
The rhythm taking me higher

And I've become of you
You become my light
Holding me from the fire
Burning away time
And though I've seemed so far away
I've never been so close
Like a castaway
I've washed upon your love

Cause I am home
And I will never leave
Now I have more
Than I will ever need
My eyes are closed
Cause in your arms I'm safe
To rest my soul
And face another day . . .

Pushed the air in and out of my lungs
Let it fall on your chest
And all that I ever loved
Found it there in your breath

And I've become of you
You become my light
Holding me from the fire
Burning away time
Though I've seemed so far away
I've never been so close
Like a castaway
I've washed upon your love

Cause I am home
And I will never leave
Now I have more
Than I will ever need
My eyes are closed
Cause in your arms I'm safe
To rest my soul
And face another day . . . Face another day . . .

SEBASTIAN KRYS
Soraya's co-producer on her fifth and final album, *El Otro Lado de Mi* (The Better Side of Me)

Soraya was ridiculously thorough and committed to everything she did. When the disease started to take more of a grip, and she slowed down some, she took up some new hobbies. I called her up one day and she was a bit out of breath. I asked her what was going on, and she said she had decided to work on a vegetable garden. I thought, "That's nice, a little garden to keep her busy." Boy, was I wrong. The next time I went by her house, she took me out back where there was a patch of land the size of a small swimming pool perfectly planted and organized. Each planting was labeled with a glazed tile she had hand-made. On each tile she had hand-painted a picture of the crop she had planted, *and in calligraphy she wrote both the scientific and the common names of each vegetable, about twenty in all. I thought what I always thought when she did something: "What a freak!" She never did anything halfway. If she learned an instrument, she mastered it completely. If you were her friend, you were her FRIEND. And if she planted a vegetable garden, her vegetables could win blue ribbons at the state fair.*

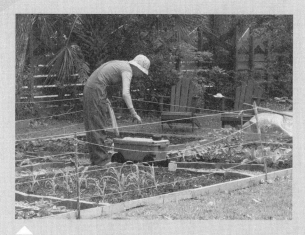

April 2006. Soraya in her garden.

ometime in April 2006, Soraya wrote a final song, called "Cannot Find My Way." Outwardly, even to those closest to her, the light of her spirit never flickered. "Music was sort of like a therapeutic thing for me," Soraya once told the *Houston Chronicle.* "I always tell people even if you can't sing or you can't paint or whatever, just find an outlet. Find something where you don't have to think, where you can just feel, and you just let it out."

> *But I feel it closing in*
> *Wonder what I could have been*
> *In another time, another place*
>
> *But I've been dealt this hand*
> *No choice but to understand*
> *Maybe I've paid my dues*
> *For next time*
>
> *—Soraya, 2006*

209

ITZEL DIAZ
Soraya's closest friend

Soraya was crazy funny, even in the late stages of her cancer. Only a week or so before she left us, she insisted on going for a ride in the car. Her mother's brother, Elciario, was in town visiting, and Soraya had bought herself a new BMW in the spring. It was a special-order 525i. She never was the type to go for the most extravagant model, but now she allowed herself the luxury, and she wanted to show it off. She pushed and prodded and got everyone in that car, including herself. I drove, and she kept looking back at Elciario with this self-satisfied look on her face like, "So there. Who has the nicer car now?" Of course it was all in fun, but here she is, in the most horrible situation imaginable, and she's ribbing her uncle about who drives a nicer car. Her spirit was absolutely unstoppable.

On May 7, Joyce showed Soraya the first typeset pages of Soraya's newly edited manuscript. Joyce wanted to give Soraya an idea of what *Broken Strings* (her book title as she intended it) might look like as a finished product. Joyce even had some sample cover art to show Soraya. This got huge smiles as Soraya realized that her dream of publishing a book to benefit the cause would be coming true.

The goodbye letter posted on her Web site May 9

The road hasn't always been easy; however, I have learned that when it comes to some things, there is no other choice than to embrace whatever path you are on. Regardless of my path, hopes, dreams, and expectations have never failed to be present. In those dreams you have been unconditional accomplices, sometimes walking by my side, singing with me or carrying my message of hope to places I have been unable to physically reach. For this, I am eternally grateful. You have given me so many gifts. I thank you for the privilege of performing for you, through my songs or at my concerts, where your applause lovingly crept into my heart. I thank you for the privilege of writing you as it brought me much clarity, and even though I have been quiet for some time, all the while, the pages of my internal diary have been active. As I have gone deeper into myself in search of my inner soul, my only truth, what I've discovered is that my spirit has been rewarded deeply by some of the stories many of you have shared with me through e-mails or letters, by some of the experiences we've had together, and also through personal thoughts that were the fruits of your generosity.

Lately, my diary pages have ceased to be internal. I've tried to share all I can, deeply and sincerely, in a new written work that I hope will be the answer to many questions that have not been elaborated on or answered as of yet. The ability to write my memoir has reinforced the fact that although material compensation is necessary for everyday living, spiritual rewards are the ones that have truly allowed me to live life, joyously in the way life is meant to be lived—where we live just for the sheer sake of living.

Thank you for opening your hearts to my music. Had you not lent me your ears, my songs would be merely dreams. My art has always been pure joy, lovingly created because of you and for you. I hope that my songs and my book will allow you to feel, think, appreciate, question, yearn, and especially, love.

My journey today is not easy. Still, as I write this, I am at peace, and everywhere around me I see and hear harmony. All is

211

as it should be because I know I am incredibly fortunate in so many ways. My dream to create music that moves people, as well as my dream to communicate a mission that would change people, have been realized. I can say with certainty that I have fulfilled my dreams, and today, I cannot ask for more. This enables me to move forward even now, with hope, and without fear.

My mission began as a dream and became a reality because of you. Today my voice is no longer a lonely cry; it grows every day through your voices. It doesn't matter whether we've had the opportunity to smile face-to-face or not, each one of you has been and will always be a blessing to me.

My physical history may come to an end, but I am confident my existence will leave its mark for the future benefit of many women. I am comforted that the light from my life will shine on many more families. Today I have not lost this battle, no pain is felt in vain, because I know my struggle will help overcome a greater battle, that of early detection and prevention against this terrible enemy. The essence of life lies in transcending through others. By offering the value of my experience and my struggles I hope to lift up many more voices. We still have not reached the goal, but I know we are closer to it every day.

Now it is up to you to continue with our mission. I hope with all my heart that my love for life has caught on and that you will become a means of communicating this message to many people whose lives may be saved. Please, recognize this opportunity you have now to stop an enemy that can end your life. Don't give up! The road ahead is long and this is a battle worth fighting.

¡No se dejen vencer! Hay mucho camino que recorrer y esta lucha vale la pena.

"When the only sound that breaks the silence is your beating heart, in between the pounding you will find who you are."

Con amor,

Soraya

he world press picked up the news and word traveled fast. Friends, fans, and those affected by Soraya's mission responded by e-mail. Soraya was awake and in control until her last breath, and her family and friends read some of the e-mails to her. Reaching the very end of her journey understanding she had touched so many lives gave her great comfort and peace.

J.J.R.
One of Soraya's many fans

Soraya . . .

Thank you for your beautiful words of inspiration. Every time I listen to your CD regarding the importance of doing a self breast exam, the hair stands up on my arms. I started the CD "Pass It Forward" message in all of the oncology offices I visit. Each person who receives your CD is encouraged to listen and pass this very important message on to another woman. I am walking in the Susan G. Komen sixty-mile "Breast Cancer Three-Day." I will walk in honor of you and all other HEROS. . . .

God Bless you and your family during this very difficult time.
With LOVE and appreciation of your beautiful voice and music.

OLGUI CHIRINO
Soraya's long-time back-up vocalist, keyboard player, and musical director

In May 2006, I was in Barcelona in production rehearsals preparing to go on tour with Shakira, another Colombian artist. One evening, I got a call from my mother, who said she needed to talk to me and it was important.

I hadn't seen Soraya in almost a year and a half. In December of 2004, while Soraya was in production for El Otro Lado De Mi, *we were asked to participate in a memorial songwriter's showcase honoring Ellen Moraskie. We were both very good friends with her so Soraya and I agreed to do the show together. We sang "Como Seria," a song we had written together. After the performance, Soraya told me she had to leave because she had an early morning* the next day. As we were saying good-bye, she told me to call her around the holidays. She wanted to get together for Christmas and do something. I said, "Of course," and then I noticed her pulling my boyfriend aside. I figured she was probably telling him to remind me to call her for the holidays. When he came back, I asked him what Soraya had told him and he said, "Nothing really. She was just talking about you." I didn't think twice about it.

Now, my mother was on the phone, telling me that La Sori was very ill. I thought maybe it was Soraya's cell count that was bad and she would probably want to try a different treatment this time. In my mind, we were going to go through the same thing we went through last time and it was going to be okay again. My mother then told me that she was on her last breaths. "No more treatment, no more anything. Everyone's just waiting now," she said.

My legs suddenly felt like Jell-O. I had to sit down. I felt a cold rush go through my body and I started crying hysterically. The next day was May 10, and in the middle of rehearsal on the front of every Web page I saw the headlines: "Singer/songwriter Soraya loses battle with cancer at age 37." I ran out and locked myself in the bathroom at the rehearsal studio. Shakira knew Soraya. She knew that Soraya and I were good friends, and she knew of her battle with cancer. She approached me and asked me what I wanted to do. I told her I needed to go home and be with Soraya's family and pay my respects. She told me to take all the time I needed and come back when I felt better. I took a plane the next day to Miami.

I attended the service for the celebration of Soraya's life and was asked to sing one of Soraya's favorite songs, "Pueblito Viejo," at her service. I feel lucky to have known her. I know she's still with me. When I got home from her memorial service, I remember telling my boyfriend that I wished Soraya's and my last words together had been more than, "Let's get together at Christmas." Remembering how Soraya had pulled him aside the last time we were together, he looked at me and said, "At least you got 'Christmas.' Her last words to me were 'If you hurt her, I'll kill you.'" Yup, she was my sister.

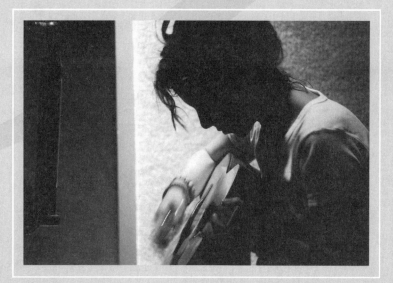

Soraya Lamilla, March 11, 1969–May 10, 2006.

Before All That

Written by Jessica Cuevas and read by her sister
Adrienne Cuevas at Soraya's memorial service

*Long before the first record contract, there was a child I knew only
from photographs. Polished and proud, smiling firmly into the
camera, this cousin of mine exuded a self-confidence not often
found in most people under the age of ten. Seeds of envy sprouted
in my heart as I gazed for extended periods at her perfect posture
and flawless skin. Meeting her for the first time, I was bemused by
the paradox of her gentle speaking voice and the intensity of her
words. How could they coexist so peacefully?*

*Long before the first recorded album there was a girl who code-
switched effortlessly from Spanish to English and back again,
depending on the company and the occasion. While other children
of first-generation immigrants hid details of their heritage for fear
of discrimination, this girl wore her cultural legacy like a badge of
honor. The traditional foods, music, customs, and language were*

215

to be celebrated, heralded, if she was going to be true to herself.

Long before the first press conference, there was a young woman with unstoppable spirit. She had the focus of a meditating yogi. Whether excelling on the soccer field, performing in the youth symphony orchestra, or maintaining the A honor roll, she pooled her energies, allowing the fountain of creativity to spew from her human form. A hand strumming deftly, a foot expertly striking a ball, words coupled with notes spilling onto a page with equal parts rhyme and reason; each was born from that searing stream of energy.

Long before the first photo shoot there was a young woman who embodied passion. She allowed herself the luxury of becoming consumed by Mozart and Beethoven, by the writings of Hemingway and Charlotte Brontë, by the hypnotic lull of the Atlantic Ocean waves. I watched her lose herself in order to find what lay within her. She trusted in the tenuous relationship between what already existed and what is yet to be formed, determined to become a living conduit between the two.

Long before the first live concert, there was a young woman who concerned herself with improving the lives of others. Without speaking, she would take the spatula from her mother and assume responsibility for turning the chicken pieces on the grill. By doing so, she allowed her mother to rest her weary legs and partake in a relaxed conversation with friends and family. The size of the gesture mattered not. What mattered was that someone's burden was eased by her actions or words.

Long before the Latin Grammy award, there was someone who knew instinctively how to dream. She was intent to conjure up life's possibilities, into shimmering, shocking configurations. She dreamt not to escape, but rather to root herself more firmly to this world. It was she who formally introduced me to the art of dreaming, a gift I am gladly obligated to share with others.

Before the first contract, album, conference, photo shoot, concert, award, there was Soraya singing to herself, summoning the splendor she would later share with all of us.

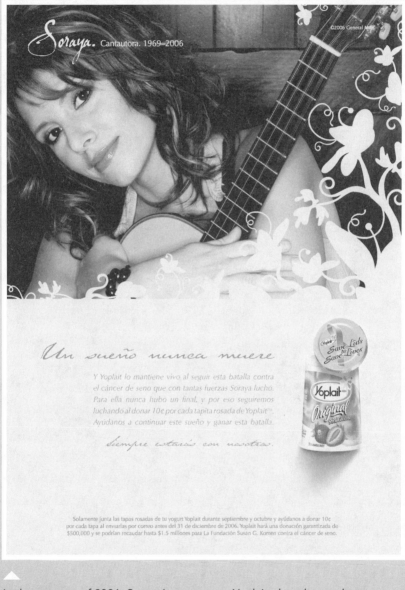

In the summer of 2006, Soraya's partners at Yoplait placed a number of tribute ads honoring the spokesperson they loved and lost. This one was headlined "A Dream Never Dies," and it talks about continuing the battle against breast cancer with the same force and energy that Soraya brought to it: "For her there was never an ending, and that's why we will keep fighting by donating ten cents for each pink lid. . . . Help us continue the dream and win this battle."

EPILOGUE

BY ITZEL DIAZ

Cowards die many times before their deaths;
The valiant never taste of death but once.
Of all the wonders that I yet have heard,
It seems to me most strange that men should fear;
Seeing that death, a necessary end,
Will come when it will come.

—William Shakespeare,
Julius Caesar, Act 2, Scene 2

In November 1995 I set up a business lunch with a new artist signed to PolyGram Records, the music company I was working for at the time. I knew very little about this artist, but having listened to her CD just days prior, I knew she was a true musician. Now, as the international marketing director for the company, I needed to see if she had the guts to make it in the music business. I had no idea I was meeting someone who was about to make such an impact on my life. The artist was Soraya. Since that day, I've been sharing her passion, determination, strength, and love for life and music. She was young, beautiful, and talented, and even then, she was determined to leave her mark in this world.

Soraya was the first bilingual artist to simultaneously release a CD in both English and Spanish—*On Nights Like This/En Esta Noche*. Island Records did the marketing for the English version and PolyGram Latin America worked the Spanish version. Success was immediate, and by the end of 1996 she had achieved superstar status. To this day, I am still amazed by her physical and mental strength. She was sheer power. The promotional tours took her to Argentina at the beginning of the week and to Germany by the weekend to perform on a TV show or some other event. She spent more time flying than being at home. She never complained, not when she fainted from sheer exhaustion in New York during the filming of one of her music videos; not when she was hospitalized in Argentina after performing with terrible acid reflux. Everyone at the record company, including myself, thought she was invincible. On her first visit to Mexico City, we went to the local market, where she bought a ring with the "S" of Superman. She never took it off. Of course the "S" stood not for Superman but for Sori, as those of close to her would call her.

One CD followed the next, as is customary in the industry, and after a lot of time on the road, we became the best of friends. But then in 2000 our Energizer Bunny fell ill. I remember the phone call from Colombia. Instantly I went from music company executive to her ally in her fight against breast cancer. I too was based in Miami, so I was able to go with her to that first appointment. As others in the music industry pondered what to do and eventually had to move on, a couple of us in her camp changed our lives and decided never to leave her side. I'm proud to say that Sori never had to go to a single doctor's appointment alone. We weathered that storm—the chemotherapy, the surgery, the radiation, and the recovery. We became a team with a mission to get healthy again, and we did.

Just as things were getting back to normal, and as irony would have it, in May 2001 I found a lump on my breast. When I told Sori, she put everything aside and became my rock. Everything that I had done for her, she now gave it back—doubled. Whereas Soraya's cancer was rare, hereditary, and very aggressive, my diagnosis was very different and in many ways much more typical of breast cancer when it's found early. I had a lumpectomy, an outpatient procedure. As a precaution, I had five rounds of chemotherapy and radiation treatments. My experience was nowhere near what Soraya had endured, but our bond grew stronger. And although she needed no further inspiration to prompt her to speak out, I can't help but think that seeing the disease strike a friend (and a friend who was also under fifty) somehow reinforced the urgency she felt. But enough about me, this is all about Sori!

In between appearances and speaking engagements, she started working on this book back in 2001. She attacked it with the same passion and tenacity as she did her music. I remember her typing away for hours. But then one day she woke up feeling really strong, and again the music and her desire to perform took hold and she wanted her career back. By early 2002 she was writing songs for her fourth album and we were working to get her a new record contract and a marketing company that would help her spread her message of early detection and hope. She recorded her new CD, and she titled it simply *Soraya*. It was a hymn of triumph—her way of shouting that she was alive and ready to face anything that came her way.

Success in the music industry is hard to achieve, but she reached the top again, which only serves to demonstrate the determination and excellence that defined Soraya. She won a Latin Grammy for Best Album by a Singer/Songwriter, competing against some of the best songwriters in Spanish language music.

Soraya started traveling again, but this time her schedule was more hectic. Along with the promotion of her CD, she had commited herself to her cause, and she had places she needed to be for the Susan G. Komen Breast Cancer Foundation, General Mills Yoplait, sanofi-aventis, and many cancer organizations throughout Latin America. She gave speeches, visited hospitals, and accompanied mammovans to grocery stores. She went anyplace where she could reach out and tell everyone that if detected early, breast cancer could be beaten. Soraya achieved more than she had ever imagined. She was writing for other artists, she was singing, she was helping the cause, and during these postdiagnosis years she even built a replica of the Colombian hacienda that her aunt America had in Cali where the family always gathered. And then . . . it happened again. The cancer came back, this time with a rage. We cried, we got mad, we asked why . . . and then, as we did before, we put on our fighting armor and faced it head-on.

This time, however, she decided to keep it private. She knew that if she made the news public, it would interfere with her music, her career, and her focus on fighting this battle. She began receiving aggressive chemotherapy treatments that made her feel worse than before, but she held up like a champion. The visits to the doctor came more often and the news was getting worse. But let's not forget that we are talking about Soraya. She continued to work. She performed, wrote new songs, put out her fifth CD (*El Otro Lado de Mi* [The Better Side of Me]), helped produce a couple of tracks for other artists, planted a world-class vegetable garden, rode her bicycle, performed big concerts, and finally finished writing this book.

In the presence of absence one tends to look at things more closely and ponder. I can write for hours on how wonderful Soraya was and how much she accomplished. But she was as human as everyone else. She always joked about the irony of being in the limelight, because she was the antithesis of a superstar. Her favorite phrase was "Be ever so humble . . ."

Her life was too short. Like me, her family, her friends, and her many, many fans feel robbed and deeply impacted by her passing. However, it must be said that she never lost faith or hope. She had bad days and good days, and she lived them to the fullest. She was a fighter. I feel honored to have been by her side until the end. I saw her take her last breath and shed her last tear. History repeated itself; she had become her mother, her *tia*, her grandmother. I sit here crying as I write these words. It was extremely hard for me to see her go.

Surrounded by her father, her uncle, her cousin, a few friends, her three dogs, and in the comfort of her own home, we saw her body being taken away. So like Sori, she stayed with us until the end. We all held hands, circled around her body, and thanked God for having shared in her life.

Then, as unbelievable as it may sound, not an hour had gone by since her last breath when this beautiful yellow bird perched atop one of the palm trees outside her room and let out a song so loud that we all looked at each other and smiled. As a songwriter Soraya was a poet, and there are numerous references in poetry and literature about the wings of birds carrying the souls of the dead up to the heavens. She had shared this thought with us, and when her cousin Bob, a birdwatcher, told us that the yellow bird was an oriole and that he had not seen one in the last five years, I wasn't surprised at all.

This world will not be the same without Soraya. Not because she is no longer with us, but because she made a difference. She left her mark. She touched many lives; she gave strength to so many people. She loved, she laughed, she cried, she knew pain, but in the end she won. She was and is a winner, even though she did not break the legacy as she had hoped. Her message was heard; her voice reached those it needed to reach. At the celebration of her life held just a couple days after her passing, a close friend told a story that described Soraya so perfectly:

A small boy went to the beach and saw the sand covered with many starfish of radiant colors. He began to pick them up one by one and throw them back in the water. A man came by and saw the boy and the thousands of starfish. He came up to the boy and told him to stop, that his effort would not make a difference. There were too many starfish to save. The boy picked up a single starfish and threw it in the ocean, saying: "I made a difference for that one."

That was Sori: if she could reach just one woman and make sure she knew about early detection, then she had made a difference. The avalanche has started. She left us all in charge of her mission. We will do everything within our power to continue her legacy, to make sure that what she wanted the most becomes a reality—to have women die *with* breast cancer, not *from* breast cancer. To let them know that if caught early, breast cancer is not a death sentence. Soraya changed my life. I will miss her physical presence, but spiritually she is right here next to me and to those who love her.

Soraya disliked thank-yous, as she was always afraid to leave someone out. But I must list a few names—Joyce, Rosie, Alison, Adri, David, Kevin, Linda, Merle, Sherry, Juliet, Loly, Jessica, Bob, Sebastian, Donna, Raul, Marya, Bilbao, Paul K., Maria, Marc S., the staff at OHG, Sandra, Vanessa, Alejandra, Cheryl, the staff at MCI-BCC, Joyce O., Nancy B., Susan C., Susan B., all the staff at Komen, and her fans.

And a special thanks to our friends at PowerPact: Rose Ann, Frenchie, Christine, Lori, Julie M., Carol, Judi, Devon, Susan G., Jenn, Melissa, Chasity, Ronda, Scott, Pierre Provost, and everyone else there. Thanks for jumping on the Soraya train and working so hard to make it go.

Gracias to all, for all the love and care you gave her.

INSPIRATIONS

ELEVEN HELPFUL THEMES

INTERPRETED AND COMPILED BY
JOYCE FLEMING AND ALISON PROVOST

Our dear friend Soraya passed away just a short time after completing this work. To one who didn't know her, it might appear senseless and sad to publish a memoir describing the immense depth and quality of her hope while living and writing, only to have her lose her life soon after finishing the work. However, to view her memoir as an exercise in futility would be to miss the point of Soraya's life and her message.

No, things did not turn out the way Soraya would have liked, nor how we and her fans would have wished. Yet it makes her message that much more poignant. What she shows us in this book is how to live—really live—whether we are healthy or dying, whether we have five years or fifty left to go.

By way of ensuring that her messages have the impact they should beyond her death, we'd like to summarize for Soraya what she could not after time ran out on her. The themes she used in her speeches, in her writings, and in this memoir have the power to enhance the quality of life and, ultimately, the meaning of a life well lived, for all of us.

Our hope is that this summary will help you benefit even more from Soraya's remarkable story.

FIND OUT WHO YOU ARE

Soraya used her battle with cancer as a road map to find her true self. Along the way she found strength she didn't know she had, a capacity to love that delighted and fulfilled her, an appreciation for everything and everyone in her life. She said, "Working our way toward a reunion with our inner self is the only accomplishment that deserves our undivided attention. It will be the fuel for all of our dreams and hopes."

What can you learn about yourself?

How can you dig deeper to live a life full of life?

DISCOVER YOUR PURPOSE

Some say we are put here for a reason, not merely to live from day to day, but to effect change for our loved ones, our neighbors, and even strangers. You can create hope in the world by as small an act as giving up your seat on a bus or a train to someone who looks tired, or as great an action as taking the time to connect with those who suffer more than you. Effecting change stems from actions, great and small. Soraya did this however and whenever she could, from kicking a soccer ball around with her nephew to tirelessly showing up to and supporting breast cancer advocacy events. She always offered hope and love.

How can you connect with your ever-changing truths and live a life worth living?

How can you discover your reason for being and use it to leave a legacy?

THEME
3

PUT YOURSELF IN CHARGE OF YOU

Many of us tend to allow others authority over our lives. Doctors are just one example; we trust their medical opinions and put ourselves in their hands. While simultaneously putting faith in her physicians, Soraya also knew that to fight cancer, to extend her life, and to live it well, she needed to act in partnership with her doctors and to be the captain navigating her own ship.

To whom have you given authority over your life?

How can you take full responsibility for where your life is going?

LISTEN CAREFULLY, AND GROW FROM WHAT YOU HEAR

It is never easy to hear bad news, let alone accept it into our lives. "Why me?" we ask. We see the dark and are tempted to tumble down into it, helpless to do anything else. But in these frightening statements of fact, there are other messages—messages that guide you toward living life to its fullest potential, messages designed to bring hope.

What good can you draw from the seemingly bad?

What messages do you think you need to hear?

THEME

5

ACCEPT YOUR REALITY AND EMBRACE IT

Soraya learned the lesson of acceptance at an early age. Her parents had little money, but they showed her how to take the current circumstance and make it the best it could be—and then some. She carried this lesson with her throughout her life, even when it meant using her diagnosis to propel a level of self-discovery that allowed her to live a fuller, more rewarding existence. She said, "I evolved beyond what I thought was my capability. Once I accepted my reality, all of the freed-up energy was channeled in another direction."

How can you embrace your reality to make your life bigger, better, and brighter right now?

ALLOW OTHERS IN TO HELP

It's odd how the simple act of accepting help can at times feel like the impossible. Allowing others to help us when we need it allows us to be loved— and to love back. It gives us strength when we need it most.

Do you wall yourself off from kind gestures and needed aid?

What might happen if you let others come in and take some of the burden off your shoulders?

THEME
7

DISCOVER YOUR OWN REASONS TO BELIEVE

Making music, looking to her *angelitos* for guidance and strength, and allowing herself to hear what the universe had to say—all of these things gave Soraya reasons to believe.

She said, "I evolved beyond what I thought was my capability. Once I accepted my reality, all of that freed-up energy was channeled in another direction."

How can you "rejoice in the possibility that all that churns inside of you will evolve you into a better person than you were just a mere few minutes ago?"

Can you feel the hope in that possibility?

THEME

8

MOVE ON, STRONGER THIS TIME

There are stories in the news every day of ordinary people doing extraordinary things. Sometimes in our lives we experience circumstances that make us believe we have used up all our resources, that we can't take another step. Soraya felt this at times, and when she did, she always managed to pick herself up, wipe away the dirt, and move along wiser, more open, and stronger than she had been the day before. You will be challenged in your life. You may be challenged right now by illness.

Can you remember a time you dealt with
devastation and how you got through it
to successfully arrive at today?

Can you once again find the strength to see
all that is still in front of you?

GIVE AND MAKE A DIFFERENCE

When you give of yourself, you reap the gold that can be gleaned only from generosity of spirit. Smile, talk, share, help, be kind—these are treasures with no price tag; these are riches that will come back to you tenfold if you open yourself up to them.

What gifts do you have that beckon to be shared?

How can you give in a way that will make a lasting difference to someone else?

BECOME YOUR OWN HERO

There are people in this world whom we admire for their beauty, their brains, their strength, their creativity. We see them and the qualities that make them extraordinary, and it is so easy to hold them in awe. But what about you? Do you know that you are strong? That you have greatness? That you have beauty that is yours and yours alone? Get up, look in the mirror, and see the hero who stands before you.

What qualities do you possess that you admire in yourself?

How can you wear these like a badge of honor?

THEME

11

PUT YOURSELF FIRST
AND LIVE A LIFE
FULL OF LIFE

In the Latina community, where women often feel that taking care of their own family must come before taking care of themselves, Soraya pointed out that the best way to take care of your family is to make sure you will be alive to do so.

We learn from Soraya to discover the moment—the importance of living a life right here and right now. Why wait until tomorrow if we can do it today?

What have you been putting off that would enrich your life if you did it today?

Have you taken the time lately to just be?

When was the last time you walked barefoot in the grass?

A MEDICAL NOTE

BY JOYCE O'SHAUGHNESSY, M.D.

Soraya's breast cancer was indeed rare, as, thankfully, breast cancer is highly uncommon in one so young. It is also uncommon for young women with breast cancer to develop a recurrence and to die of breast cancer in their thirties. With early detection and state-of-the-art treatment, about 80 to 85 percent of women diagnosed with breast cancer today will either be cured of their disease or will live for decades without evidence of disease.

And advancements are coming quickly now. Since Soraya was first diagnosed with breast cancer, our ability to detect breast cancer at a very early stage in high-risk young women with a family history of breast cancer has improved remarkably. So has our ability to increase the cure rate with improved chemotherapies, anti-HER2 antibody therapy, and antiestrogen therapies. Since 1990, every year has brought about significant advances in the early detection of breast cancer, genetic testing for hereditary predisposition, and, most important, treatment for those who are diagnosed. Even prevention of the disease is something on our horizon.

The death rate from breast cancer in the United States has been falling steadily since the mid-nineties as these advances have been put into practice. Unfortunately, Soraya's cancer was highly unusual in its ability to escape eradication despite the aggressive treatments she received. Yet I was astonished by Soraya's equanimity throughout her breast cancer journey. It seemed to me she had an understanding of life far beyond her years, as though she had already lived a complete and full existence and could float on the waves of uncertainty with courage and grace.

Soraya was very dedicated to making women aware of the threat of breast cancer and felt passionately about having her experiences benefit other women. She often spoke about trusting one's instincts regarding any changes in your breasts, being empowered and persistent when seeking medical evaluation, and of course, getting yearly mammograms at forty and older. These are words to live by.

Her messages personalized so much for all of us who marveled at her musical magic, her integrity, and her transcendent spirit.

PHOTO CREDITS